Soft and Hard Tissue Regeneration

Soft and Hard Tissue Regeneration

Special Issue Editors

Carlos E. Nemcovsky
Miron Weinreb

MDPI • Basel • Beijing • Wuhan • Barcelona • Belgrade • Manchester • Tokyo • Cluj • Tianjin

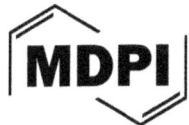

Special Issue Editors
Carlos E. Nemcovsky
Tel Aviv University
Israel

Miron Weinreb
Tel Aviv University
Israel

Editorial Office
MDPI
St. Alban-Anlage 66
4052 Basel, Switzerland

This is a reprint of articles from the Special Issue published online in the open access journal *Dentistry Journal* (ISSN 2304-6767) (available at: https://www.mdpi.com/journal/dentistry/special_issues/tissue_regeneration).

For citation purposes, cite each article independently as indicated on the article page online and as indicated below:

LastName, A.A.; LastName, B.B.; LastName, C.C. Article Title. *Journal Name* **Year**, *Article Number*, Page Range.

ISBN 978-3-03928-304-0 (Pbk)
ISBN 978-3-03928-305-7 (PDF)

© 2020 by the authors. Articles in this book are Open Access and distributed under the Creative Commons Attribution (CC BY) license, which allows users to download, copy and build upon published articles, as long as the author and publisher are properly credited, which ensures maximum dissemination and a wider impact of our publications.

The book as a whole is distributed by MDPI under the terms and conditions of the Creative Commons license CC BY-NC-ND.

Contents

About the Special Issue Editors vii

Carlos E. Nemcovsky and Miron Weinreb
Soft and Hard Tissue Regeneration—A Special Issue of Dentistry Journal
Reprinted from: *Dent. J.* **2018**, *6*, 4, doi:10.3390/dj6010004 1

José Luis Calvo-Guirado, José Eduardo Maté-Sánchez de Val, María Luisa Ramos-Oltra Carlos Pérez-Albacete Martínez, María Piedad Ramírez-Fernández, Manuel Maiquez-Gosálvez, Sergio A Gehrke, Manuel Fernández-Domínguez, Georgios E. Romanos and Rafael Arcesio Delgado-Ruiz
The Use of Tooth Particles as a Biomaterial in Post-Extraction Sockets. Experimental Study in Dogs
Reprinted from: *Dent. J.* **2018**, *6*, 12, doi:10.3390/dj6020012 3

Minas Leventis, George Agrogiannis, Peter Fairbairn, Orestis Vasiliadis, Danai Papavasileiou, Evangelia Theodoropoulou, Robert Horowitz and Demos Kalyvas
Evaluation of an In Situ Hardening β-Tricalcium Phosphate Graft Material for Alveolar Ridge Preservation. A Histomorphometric Animal Study in Pigs
Reprinted from: *Dent. J.* **2018**, *6*, 27, doi:10.3390/dj6030027 15

Stephen K. Harrel
Videoscope-Assisted Minimally Invasive Surgery (VMIS) for Bone Regeneration around Teeth and Implants: A Literature Review and Technique Update
Reprinted from: *Dent. J.* **2018**, *6*, 30, doi:10.3390/dj6030030 27

Carlos E. Nemcovsky and Ilan Beitlitum
Combination Therapy for Reconstructive Periodontal Treatment in the Lower Anterior Area: Clinical Evaluation of a Case Series
Reprinted from: *Dent. J.* **2018**, *6*, 50, doi:10.3390/dj6040050 39

Zvi Artzi, Shiran Sudri, Ori Platner and Avital Kozlovsky
Regeneration of the Periodontal Apparatus in Aggressive Periodontitis Patients
Reprinted from: *Dent. J.* **2019**, *7*, 29, doi:10.3390/dj7010029 51

Tetsuhiro Tsujino, Kazushige Isobe, Hideo Kawabata, Hachidai Aizawa, Sadahiro Yamaguchi, Yutaka Kitamura, Hideo Masuki, Taisuke Watanabe, Hajime Okudera, Koh Nakata and Tomoyuki Kawase
Spectrophotometric Determination of the Aggregation Activity of Platelets in Platelet-Rich Plasma for Better Quality Control
Reprinted from: *Dent. J.* **2019**, *7*, 61, doi:10.3390/dj7020061 65

About the Special Issue Editors

Carlos E. Nemcovsky graduated from Dental School in Montevideo, Uruguay in 1979. Post-graduate studies in Periodontology at Tel-Aviv University. Specialist in Periodontology since 1997. Full Professor at the Department of Periodontology and Implant Dentistry, The Maurice and Gabriela Goldschleger School of Dental Medicine, Tel-Aviv University Former President of the Israel Periodontal and Osseointegration Society. Author or co-author of over 100 scientific publications (most of them listed in Pubmed.org) in the leading international journals in the fields of dental research, occlusion, oral rehabilitation, periodontology and dental implants and numerous chapters in academic books. Co-editor of books: "Evidence-Based Decision Making in Dentistry. Multidisciplinary Management of the Natural Dentition" (Springer International Publishing, Switzerland, 2017) and "Endodontic-Periodontal Lesions. Evidence-Based Multidisciplinary Clinical Management" (Springer International Publishing Switzerland, 2019). Involved in basic and clinical research, with main interest in tissue regeneration. Reviewer and member of the editorial boards for several scientific journals. Well-renowned international speaker, with over 120 invited lectures in addition to numerous presentations at scientific meetings worldwide and continuing education courses in the fields of periodontology and dental implants. Holds a private practice limited to periodontics and dental implants.

Miron Weinreb is a full Professor in the Department of Oral Biology, Goldschleger School of Dental Medicine, Tel-Aviv University in Israel. He earned his D.M.D. degree from the Hadassah School of Dental Medicine of the Hebrew University in Jerusalem, Israel and spent his post-doctoral training in the Department of Bone Biology and Osteoporosis, Merck Research Laboratories in West-Point, PA, USA. His main research interests are the effects of systemic diseases, mainly diabetes, on the skeleton and on periodontal regeneration and the cellular effects of prostaglandins in the gingival and bone tissues. He has published ¿90 research papers in peer-reviewed journals.

Preface to "Soft and Hard Tissue Regeneration"

The continuous presence of bacteria at the tooth–epithelium or implant–epithelium junction results in a progressive inflammatory process, which leads to the destruction of the gingival connective tissue and subsequently of the alveolar bone, periodontal ligament (PDL) and cementum on the root and/or implant surface. If left undisturbed, this process will eventually lead to the loss of the tooth or implant. However, this loss of periodontal support is not only detrimental to the stability and function of the tooth or implant; it also largely complicates the restoration of the diseased area with implants following the removal of the affected tooth/implant. Accordingly, great attention has been paid to periodontal and bone reconstructive treatment.

In the field of bone regeneration, the determination of the aggregation activity of platelets in platelet-rich plasma [1] suggests that the spectrophotometric method may be useful in quick chair-side evaluation of individual PRP quality.

A novel in situ hardening β-tricalcium phosphate graft material for alveolar ridge preservation and tooth particles were evaluated in two different animal studies [2,3].

A videoscope-assisted minimally invasive surgery (VMIS) for bone regeneration around teeth and implants was thoroughly reviewed, together with a technique update [4].

In the field of periodontal reconstructive treatment, an extensive review on the topic of regeneration of the periodontal apparatus in aggressive periodontitis patients and a clinical evaluation of a case series that was treated with a combination therapy for reconstructive periodontal treatment in the lower anterior area are also included [5,6].

Carlos E. Nemcovsky, Miron Weinreb
Guest Editors

References

1. Tsujino, T.; Isobe, K.; Kawabata, H.; Aizawa, H.; Yamaguchi, S.; Kitamura, Y.; Masuki, H.; Watanabe, T.; Okudera, H.; Nakata, K.; et al. Spectrophotometric Determination of the Aggregation Activity of Platelets in Platelet-Rich Plasma for Better Quality Control. *Dent. J.* **2019**, *7*, 61.
2. Leventis, M.; Agrogiannis, G.; Fairbairn, P.; Vasiliadis, O.; Papavasileiou, D.; Theodoropoulou, E.; Horowitz, R.; Kalyvas, D. Evaluation of an In Situ Hardening β-Tricalcium Phosphate Graft Material for Alveolar Ridge Preservation. A Histomorphometric Animal Study in Pigs. *Dent. J.* **2018**, *6*, 27.
3. Calvo-Guirado, J.L.; Maté-Sánchez de Val, J.E.; Ramos-Oltra, M.L.; Pérez-Albacete Martínez, C.; Ramírez-Fernández, M.P.; Maiquez-Gosálvez, M.; Gehrke, S.A.; Fernández-Domínguez, M.; Romanos, G.E.; Delgado-Ruiz, R.A. The Use of Tooth Particles as a Biomaterial in Post-Extraction Sockets. Experimental Study in Dogs. *Dent. J.* **2018**, *6*, 12.
4. Artzi, Z.; Sudri, S.; Platner, O.; Kozlovsky, A. Regeneration of the Periodontal Apparatus in Aggressive Periodontitis Patients. *Dent. J.* **2019**, *7*, 29.
5. Nemcovsky, C.E.; Beitlitum, I. Combination Therapy for Reconstructive Periodontal Treatment in the Lower Anterior Area: Clinical Evaluation of a Case Series. *Dent. J.* **2018**, *6*, 50.

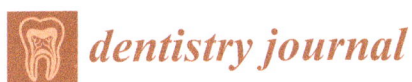

Editorial

Soft and Hard Tissue Regeneration—A Special Issue of Dentistry Journal

Carlos E. Nemcovsky [1,*] and Miron Weinreb [2]

1. Department of Periodontology and Dental Implantology, Goldschleger School of Dental Medicine, Tel Aviv University, Tel-Aviv 69978, Israel
2. Department of Oral Biology, Goldschleger School of Dental Medicine, Tel Aviv University, Tel-Aviv 69978, Israel; weinreb@post.tau.ac.il
* Correspondence: carlos@post.tau.ac.il

Received: 25 December 2017; Accepted: 17 January 2018; Published: 23 January 2018

This Special Issue entitled "Soft and Hard Tissue Regeneration" will cover both periodontal and implant therapies.

The goal of regenerative periodontal treatment is to restore functional periodontal support offering a valuable treatment alternative even for teeth with large periodontal destruction. With successful treatment, these may be successfully maintained in health for long periods. In most cases where teeth are extracted for periodontal reasons, implant therapy will demand an intermediate bone augmentation procedure. Thus, lack of sufficient bone volume may prevent placement of dental implants.

Although most bone grafts are only able to fill and maintain a space, where bone regeneration can occur ("osteoconductive"), the ideal bone graft will also promote bone production and hence osseous regeneration ("osteoinductive").

Several bone augmentation procedures have been described, each presenting advantages and shortcomings.

The success of bone augmentation procedures depends on the presence of bone forming cells, primary wound closure over the augmented area, space creation and maintenance where bone can grow, and proper angiogenesis of the grafted area.

Factors that influence the choice of the surgical technique are the estimated duration of surgical procedure, its complexity, cost, total estimated length of procedure until the final rehabilitation may be installed, and the surgeons' experience.

This Special Issue will have a definite clinical orientation, and will be entirely dedicated to soft and hard tissue regenerative treatment alternatives, both in periodontal and in implant therapy, discussing their rationale, indications and clinical procedures. Internationally-renowned leading researchers and clinicians will contribute with articles in their field of expertise.

Keywords

- periodontal treatment
- dental implants
- orthodontic treatment
- complications
- pre-clinical research
- clinical research
- esthetics
- maxillary sinus
- bone augmentation
- bone grafts
- membranes

- osteoconduction
- osteoinduction
- growth factors
- therapy

Conflicts of Interest: The authors declare no conflict of interest.

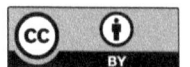 © 2018 by the authors. Licensee MDPI, Basel, Switzerland. This article is an open access article distributed under the terms and conditions of the Creative Commons Attribution (CC BY) license (http://creativecommons.org/licenses/by/4.0/).

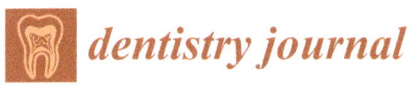

Article

The Use of Tooth Particles as a Biomaterial in Post-Extraction Sockets. Experimental Study in Dogs

José Luis Calvo-Guirado [1,*], José Eduardo Maté-Sánchez de Val [1], María Luisa Ramos-Oltra [1], Carlos Pérez-Albacete Martínez [1], María Piedad Ramírez-Fernández [2], Manuel Maiquez-Gosálvez [3], Sergio A Gehrke [4], Manuel Fernández-Domínguez [5], Georgios E. Romanos [6] and Rafael Arcesio Delgado-Ruiz [7]

1. Faculty of Health Sciences, Universidad Católica de Murcia (UCAM), Campus de los Jerónimos N° 135, Guadalupe, 30107 Murcia, Spain; jemate@ucam.edu (J.E.M.-S.d.V.); mlramos@ucam.edu (M.L.R.-O.); cperezalbacete@ucam.edu (C.P.-A.M.)
2. Department of Epidemiology, Universidad Católica de Murcia (UCAM), 30107 Murcia, Spain; mpramirez@ucam.edu
3. Faculty of Health Sciences, Department of Oral and Implant Dentistry Universidad Católica de Murcia (UCAM), 30107 Murcia, Spain; sergio.gehrke@hotmail.com
4. Biotecnos Research Center—Tecnología e Ciencia Ltd., 11100 Montevideo, Uruguay; sergio.gehrke@hotmail.com
5. Faculty of Dentistry, Department of Oral and Implant Dentistry, San Pablo University CEU, Group HM (Hospital Madrid), 28050 Madrid, Spain; clinferfun@yahoo.es
6. Department of Periodontology, School of Dental Medicine, Stony Brook University, New York, 11794 NY, USA; Georgios.Romanos@stonybrookmedicine.edu
7. Department of Prosthodontics and Digital Technology, School of Dental Medicine, Stony Brook University, New York, 11794 NY, USA; Rafael.Delgado-Ruiz@stonybrookmedicine.edu
* Correspondence: jlcalvo@ucam.edu; Tel.: +34-670-785208 or +34-968-268353

Received: 30 January 2018; Accepted: 2 May 2018; Published: 6 May 2018

Abstract: Objectives: The objective of this study was to evaluate new bone formation derived from freshly crushed extracted teeth, grafted immediately in post-extraction sites in an animal model, compared with sites without graft filling, evaluated at 30 and 90 days. **Material and Methods**: The bilateral premolars P2, P3, P4 and the first mandibular molar were extracted atraumatically from six Beagle dogs. The clean, dry teeth were ground immediately using the Smart Dentin Grinder. The tooth particles obtained were subsequently sieved through a special sorting filter into two compartments; the upper container isolating particles over 1200 µm, the lower container isolated particles over 300 µm. The crushed teeth were grafted into the post-extraction sockets at P3, P4 and M1 (test group) (larger and smaller post-extraction alveoli), while P2 sites were left unfilled and acted as a control group. Tissue healing and bone formation were evaluated by histological and histomorphometric analysis after 30 and 90 days. **Results**: At 30 days, test site bone formation was greater in the test group than the control group ($p < 0.05$); less immature bone was observed in the test group (25.71%) than the control group (55.98%). At 90 days, significant differences in bone formation were found with more in the test group than the control group. No significant differences were found in new bone formation when comparing the small and large alveoli post-extraction sites. **Conclusions**: Tooth particles extracted from dog's teeth, grafted immediately after extractions can be considered a suitable biomaterial for socket preservation.

Keywords: Smart Dentin Grinder; tooth particles; autogenous particulate tooth graft; socket preservation; dog study

1. Introduction

There is compelling evidence that immediate grafting of extraction sockets using various ridge preservation techniques—including the placement of graft materials and/or the use of occlusive membranes—will prevent alveolar bone loss during the repair phase of wound healing. However, the technique lacks the capacity to promote osteogenesis and osteoinduction, and so its usefulness is limited in terms of the formation of viable bone [1].

Human demineralized dentin matrix created from extracted human teeth was first developed in 2008 and its use in implant dentistry has been evaluated on the basis of its osteoinductive, osteoconductive, and remodeling capacity. By weight, dentin and bone are composed of 30% collagen, 60% hydroxyapatite, and 10% body fluid [2–5]; by volume, they are composed of 10% liquid, 20% collagen, and 70% hydroxyapatite. These proportions place bone and dentin in the same class of material as biomaterials that consist of collagen and ceramic material [6–10].

Kim and his team have been investigating the development of biomaterials using human teeth since 1993, and have recently reported the promising results of their research [11–17]. Tooth dentin and cementum structure are similar to membranous bone in their mineral and protein composition; when new bone matrix is directly deposited on membranous surfaces, this results in ankylosed dentin-bone interfaces [18,19]. When avulsed teeth are re-implanted back into their sockets or when extracted teeth are processed immediately after being extracted into a particulate dentin graft that is inserted into freshly extracted socket in the same patient, this also creates ankylosed interfaces [20–22].

The "Smart Dentin Grinder"™ device has been designed to crush and sort extracted teeth into tooth particles of specific sizes. A chemical cleanser and a buffer are applied for 15–20 mins to eliminate bacteria. This novel procedure can be indicated for most tooth extractions, although endodontically treated teeth are counter-indicated due to contamination by foreign materials.

The objective of this study was to evaluate immature bone and new bone formation after filling fresh extraction sockets in an animal model with tooth particle graft compared with empty sockets, after a 90-day follow-up.

2. Material and Methods

Six Beagle dogs about one year old, weighing 14–15 kg each were used in the study. The University of Murcia Ethics Committee for Animal Research approved the study protocol A1320140404 (12-02-2015), which followed guidelines established by the Directive of the Council of the European Union of February 1, 2013/53/CEE, guidelines for animal studies.

The animals were quarantined for the application of rabies and vitamin vaccines. The animals were kept in cages before and after the operation and received appropriate veterinary attention during the study period. All the animals presented intact dental arches, without viral or fungal mouth lesions.

The animals were pre-anesthetized with 10% zolazepam at 0.10 mL/kg and acepromazine maleate (Calmo-Neosan®, Pfizer, Madrid, Spain) 0.12–0.25 mg/kg and medetomidine 35 mg/kg (Medetor 1 mg, Virbac, CP-Pharma Hand-elsgesellschaft GmbH, Burgdorf, Germany). The mixture was injected intramuscularly into the quadriceps femoris. The animals were taken to the operating theatre where, at the first opportunity, an intravenous catheter (diameter 22 G or 20 G) was inserted into the cephalic vein, and propofol infusion was administered at a rate of 0.4 mg/kg/min at a constant infusion rate.

Anesthetic maintenance was performed with volatile anesthetics and the animals underwent tracheal intubation with a Magill probe for the adaptation of the anesthetic device and for the administration of volatile isoflurane diluted in oxygen (2 V%). In addition, local anesthesia (Articaine 40 mg, 1% epinephrine, Normon®, Madrid, Spain) was administered at the surgical sites. These procedures were carried out under the supervision of a veterinary surgeon.

Mandibular premolars and first molars (P2, P3, P4, M1) were extracted bilaterally (Figure 1) under general anesthesia.

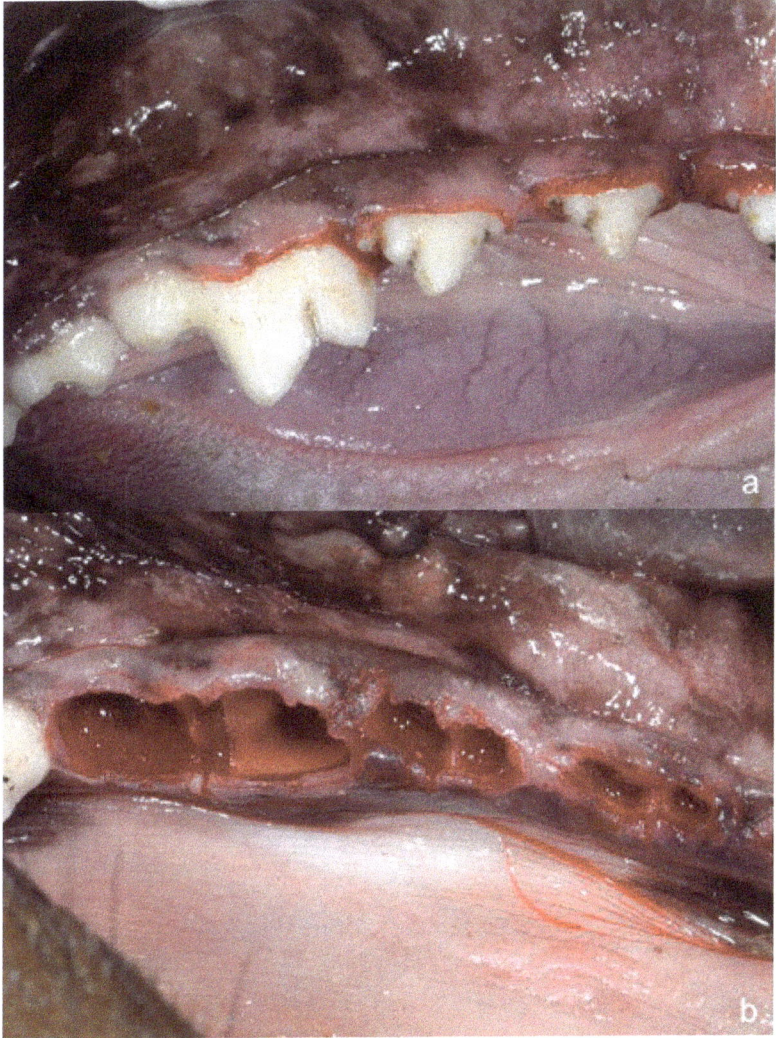

Figure 1. (**a**) Bilateral mandibular premolars P2, P3, P4 and first molar to be extracted; (**b**) Post-extraction sockets of mandibular premolars and first molars.

Teeth with multiple roots were hemisectioned in bucco-lingual direction, protecting the remaining bony walls. Immediately after extraction, the clinician eliminated the organic coating of the root surfaces that includes periodontal ligament tissue and bacterial biofilm, which was removed using a tungsten carbide bur, or hand-piece drill and water.

The teeth were cleaned, dried with an airflow syringe, and crushed immediately after extraction isolating the crown and root using the "Smart Dentin Grinder" (Bioner Sistemas Implantológicos, Barcelona, Spain), specially designed for this procedure. The tooth particles obtained were sized at 300–1200 µm, which were sieved through a special sorting system into two compartments: the upper container has a grid to isolate larger particles of over 1200 µm, while the lower container is more rigid, allowing the accumulation of smaller particles of over 300 µm (Figure 2).

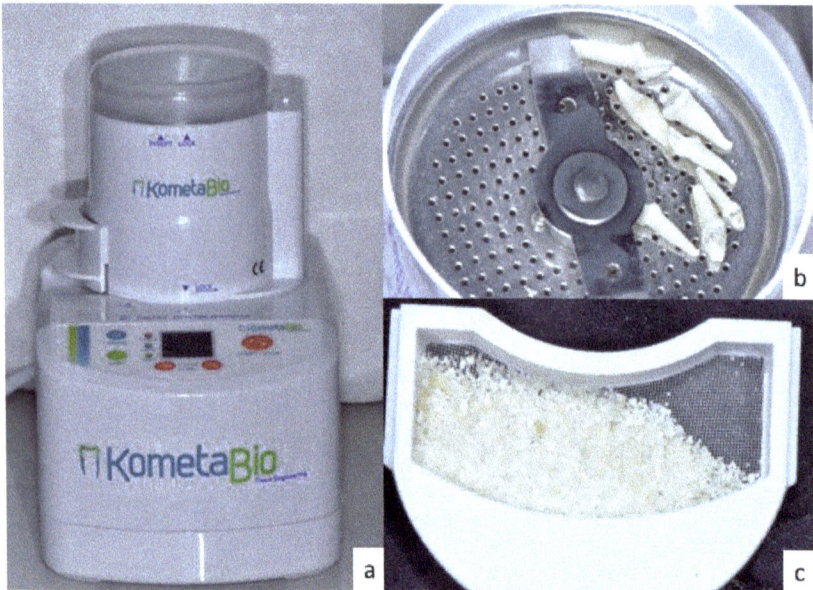

Figure 2. (a) Smart dentin grinder device; (b) Dog's extracted premolar teeth inside grinding chamber; (c) Tooth particles of 300–1200 microns obtained after using the grinding device.

More than 95% of the tooth particulate accumulates in a sterile "drawer chamber" that isolates particles of 300–1200 μm (the optimal size for achieving an osteogenic interaction at the grafted site), isolating smaller and larger particles in separate trays. The particulate volume is about 2–3 times greater than the original volume of the tooth. The particle size criteria is based on the fact that small particles facilitate quick bone resorption (300 μm) and bone maintenance, while larger particles (over 1200 μm) protect against and reduce bone resorption. Both type of tooth particles were obtained in two different compartments and the proportion of both particles used were 80% of big particles and 20% of small particles to avoid inflammation.

The particulate teeth were immersed in a basic alcohol cleanser in a sterile container for 15 min to dissolve all organic waste and bacteria. The particles were then washed with sterile saline for 5 min. Then the particles were dried, and the small and large tooth particles were mixed. The particulate was then grafted into post-extraction sites of premolars P3, P4 and first molar M1 (test group), they were filled with freshly extracted teeth (Figure 3), while the premolar P2 sockets on both sides remained unfilled, acting as control sites.

Ethanol 70% denatures and precipitates proteins and so is bactericidal. The present experiment used a 30% solution of 70% ethanol, which, in addition to its main bactericidal action, strongly enhances the action of NaOH, which eliminates organic compounds, while ethanol does not. So, the combination of ethanol and NaOH completely dissolves every organic substance and acts as a very effective disinfectant. Ethanol only affects organic compounds on the outside surface of the mineral (external organic substances). It does not penetrate the mineral and so does not affect collagen trapped in the mineral itself (which, in any case, is not infected).

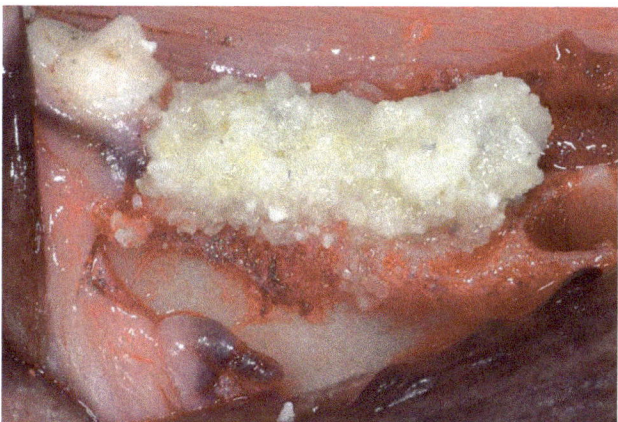

Figure 3. Ground tooth particles filling P3, P4 and first Molar M1 sockets. No material was placed into premolar P2 sockets, which acted as control sites.

Continuous non-absorbable sutures (Silk 3.0, Lorca Marin, Lorca, Murcia, Spain) were used to protect and maintain the grafted areas (Figure 4). The stitches were removed after 15 days.

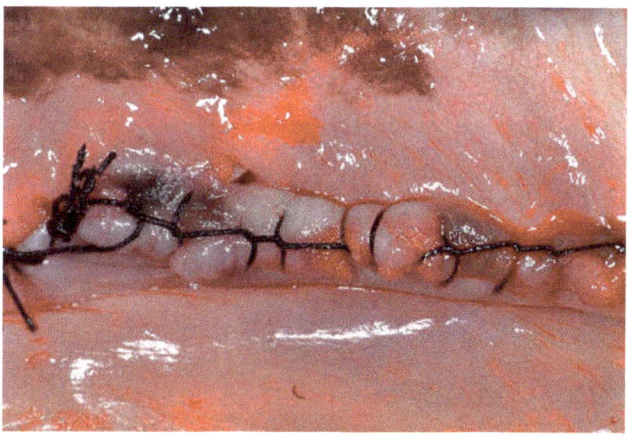

Figure 4. Continuous non-absorbable sutures (Silk 3.0, Lorca Marin, Lorca, Murcia, Spain) were used to protect and maintain the grafted areas.

Mandibular teeth from canine to canine were maintained and no surgeries were performed in the upper maxilla. All surgical techniques were performed under the supervision of the University veterinarian, assigned to the University of Murcia's Animal Research Unit.

During the surgical procedure, the animals were hydrated with glucose-saline (250 cm^3) to aid post-surgical recovery. Following the guidelines established by the animal research ethics committees, anti-inflammatory and antibiotic drugs were administered after surgery and every other day for seven days to prevent postoperative infection and inflammation: the anti-inflammatory, Metacam®(Boehringer, Ingelheim Vetmedica, Ingelheim, Germany), 1–2 mL intramuscularly; and the antibiotic Alsir®(enrofloxacin), 2 mL intramuscularly.

After surgery, the dogs were transferred to individual cages where they remained under veterinary supervision. The animals were fed ad-libitum with a soft diet during the study period.

The animals' soft tissues were disinfected and cleaned with a mouthwash based on seawater: Sea 4 Encías (Blue Sea Laboratories, Alicante, Spain).

After 30 and 90 days healing, a local anesthetic was applied to the buccal and lingual gums and crestal incisions were made in the area regenerated from the canine to the second molar (Figure 5). A full thickness mucoperiosteal flap was lifted and, using a 3 mm diameter trephine bur, biopsies were extracted from the control sites and from the areas of regenerated bone on both sides of the mandible (Figure 6).

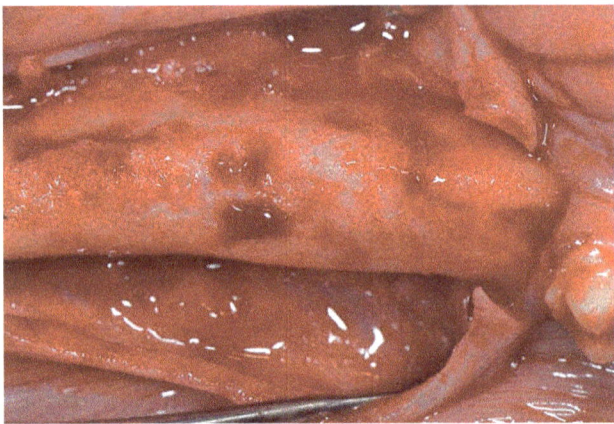

Figure 5. Healing bone in regenerated area at 90 days.

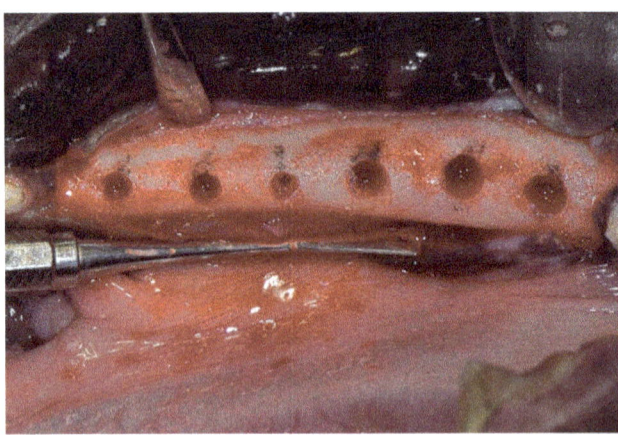

Figure 6. Core sites of tooth particles and control sites at 90 days.

2.1. Histology

The bone cores obtained were individually preserved in 10% formaldehyde for 20 days. The samples were then decalcified for 30 days using TBD-2 (Anatomical Pathology International, Runcorn, Cheshire, UK). After dehydration and inclusion in paraffin, sections of 20 μm thickness were prepared; samples were stained with picrosirius-hematoxylin and hematoxylin to distinguish between immature and mature bone.

For histomorphometric analysis, images were enlarged 20×, and eight fields per sample were evaluated digitally (using a DP12 digital camera, Olympus, Nagano, Japan). Microimage 4.0 software (Media Cybernetics, Silver Spring, MD, USA) was used for image analysis.

All analyses were carried out by the same technician, who was blinded to each sample's group assignation (test or control).

The total area of newly formed bone and connective tissue were evaluated and the percentage of immature bone was measured.

2.2. Statistical Analysis

Statistical analysis was performed using SPSS 21.0 software (SPSS, Chicago, IL, USA). Descriptive statistics were calculated (mean and standard deviation) for both groups. For the comparison of means, a non-parametric Friedman test was applied with a significance level of 95% ($p < 0.05$). The Mann–Whitney U test, a non-parametric test, was applied and the ANOVA test was used to analyze the differences between variables.

3. Results

Sample sizes were 3.5 mm in diameter by 8.5 mm in length (6 alveolus per dog) and 6 mm by 10 mm length (2 alveolus per dog) a total of 36 small and 12 big alveolus filled for both test and control specimens.

3.1. Histological Analysis at 30 Days

Control samples showed large amounts of newly formed immature bone covering the bone defect, and highly disorganized tissues with high rates of cellularity and large medullary cavities.

The tooth particulate group showed newly formed bone with irregular disposition and high levels of capillarity, but to a lesser extent than the control group (Figure 7a,b).

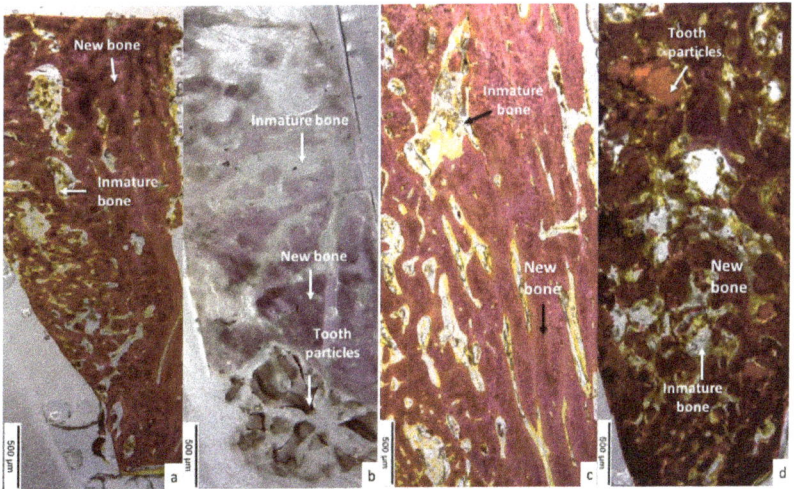

Figure 7. (a) Control group showed large quantity of newly formed immature formed bone covering the bone defect; (b) tooth particle group samples were characterized by the presence of newly formed bone of irregular disposition, with high levels of cellularity (test group); (c) images show newly formed osteons with non-organized immature bone in the control group at 90 days; (d) tooth particle group (test group) showing newly formed well organized mature bone at 90 days.

3.2. Histomorphometric Evaluation

At 30 days, new bone formation was 72.35 ± 0.98% in the defects treated with tooth particle grafts (test group), while in the untreated defects (control group) new bone formation was 55.87 ± 0.32%, with statistically significant difference between the groups ($p < 0.05$) (Table 1).

Table 1. Mean values ± standard deviation of new bone and connective tissue quantity at 30 days statistically significant difference ($p < 0.05$)*.

Evaluation at 30 Days	Tooth Particulate Mean ± SD % Test Group	Control Group	p-Value
New bone	72.35 ± 0.98 *	55.87 ± 0.32	<0.011 *
Connective tissue	22.82 ± 0.54	31.76 ± 0.61	<0.791

* statistically significant difference ($p < 0.05$).

At 90 days, new bone was 77.18 ± 0.76% in defects treated with tooth particle grafts (test group), compared with the control group (58.92 ± 0.32%) with statistically significant difference ($p < 0.05$)*. (Table 2).

Table 2. Mean values ± standard deviation of new bone formation and connective tissue at 90 days ($p < 0.05$).

Evaluation at 90 Days	Tooth Particulate Mean ± SD %	Control	p-Value
New bone	77.18 ± 0.76	59.92 ± 0.32	<0.017 *
Connective tissue	10.68 ± 0.42	22.89 ± 0.27	<0.561

* statistically significant difference ($p < 0.05$).

3.3. Histological Analysis at 90 Days

The control group showed greater bone organization compared with the 30-day evaluation. All bone defects were completely covered by newly formed osteons, while other areas were occupied by non-organized immature bone (Figure 7c). The test group showed mature newly formed bone, well organized by multiple osteons throughout the entire bone (Figure 7d).

3.4. Histomorphometric Evaluation of Immature Bone

At 30 days, histomorphometric analysis found immature bone (25.71 ± 0.25%) in defects treated with tooth particulate with significant difference between the test and control groups (55.98 ± 0.16%). At 90 days, histomorphometric analysis found total immature bone of 14.2 ± 0.66% in the test group with significant differences in comparison with the control group (35.17 ± 0.74%) (Table 3).

Table 3. Mean values ± standard deviation of the quantity of immature bone quantity at 30 and 90 days ($p < 0.05$)*.

	Quantity OF Immature Bone	
	Tooth Particulate (%) Mean ± SD Test Group	Control (%) Mean ± SD Control Group
30 days	25.71 ± 0.25 *	55.98 ± 0.16
90 days	14.2 ± 0.66 *	35.17 ± 0.74

* statistically significant difference ($p < 0.05$).

4. Discussion

Our last published work described how fresh extraction sockets can be grafted with tooth particles made by crushing the extracted teeth; bone formation was evaluated after 30 days and 90 days (the early stages of healing) finding more immature and mature bone at test sites than control sites at both study times 22). Although in the present study, the statistical method was different, the present results were similar to the earlier study, observing more immature bone at 30 days and more mature bone at 90 days, with less connective tissue. These data show how the tooth particles resorb and are replaced by new bone at 90 days.

Teeth that suffer trauma have ankylosed roots, which continuously resorb over time and are replaced by bone, eventually resorbing the entire root, while the alveolar bone is conserved during this period. Malmgren et al. described the decoronation method, offering possible explanations for the favorable outcome of this technique and proposing guidelines for deciding the correct time for intervention. After decoronation, the alveolar ridge was maintained in buccal/palatal direction, and the bone level increased, so maintaining normal alveolar conditions [23]. Pang et al. used autogenous demineralized dentin matrix from extracted teeth to graft extraction sockets and augment the vertical dimension; this was found to be as effective as augmentation using an organic bovine bone [24].

The present results reveal a close and direct interaction between mineralized dentin, bone matrix, and the grafted tooth particle material. When the extraction of a tooth is necessary, the Smart Dentin Grinder makes it possible to prepare the tooth particles from the freshly extracted autologous tooth, ready for use in as little as 15 min during a single surgical session. With no antigenicity, it improves bone remodeling capabilities and can be considered a viable graft option given its autogenous origin and favorable clinical and histological results. Moreover, despite its inductive properties, mineralized dentin integrates into newly formed bone, creating a stable site for dental implant insertion. In fact, several clinical studies have shown that implant insertion and loading can be performed in both upper and lower jaws as early as 2–4 months after grafting with crushed and demineralized tooth and bone [25,26].

Since mineralized dentin is remodeled very slowly, as compared with cortical bone, the aesthetic and structural integrity of the alveolar ridge is maintained for many years [27,28]. The patient's tooth is comparable to autogenous bone graft material and possesses all the properties of the patient´s bone due to its very similar components to bone, making it very useful in many clinical situations. The teeth and the jaw have a high level of affinity, with similar physical, chemical structures and composition [24].Kim et al. reported that 90% of the organic component of the tooth are type I collagen, which is very important in bone calcification [27–32].

Autogenous demineralized dentin matrix from extracted tooth grafted to extraction sockets for the augmentation of vertical dimension was as effective as augmentation using anorganic bovine bone. Both groups showed favorable wound healing, similar amount of implant stability, and histologically confirmed new bone formation. Thus, the results of this study suggest that autogenous tooth graft material is a viable option for alveolar bone augmentation following dental extraction [33].

It also overcomes patients' rejection of materials derived from animal or synthetic sources, as well as providing excellent biocompatibility without provoking an immune response, foreign material reaction, or infection. Unless it is contaminated by an infectious lesion, a tooth does not cause problems, even when the root tip is left in the alveolar bone. The use of the patient's own tooth is entirely legal, providing the patient agrees.

In the present study, the crushed tooth particulate produced more bone regeneration at 90 days than control samples. As the dentin graft maintains the collagen structure, it preserves both the height and width of bone crests.

5. Conclusions

Within the limitations of the present animal study, it would appear that tooth particle graft (both enamel and dentin) can be viewed as a useful autogenous biomaterial for socket preservation due to its similar characteristics to autologous bone. Currently, this graft material can be used in combination with autologous bone debris as an excellent graft material without compromising the capacity for bone regeneration.

Author Contributions: For research articles with several authors, a short paragraph specifying their individual contributions must be provided. The following statements should be used "Conceptualization, Jose Luis Calvo-Guirado; Methodology, José Eduardo Maté-Sánchez de Val, Manuel Maiquez-Gosálvez; Software, María Luisa Ramos-Oltra; Validation, Carlos Pérez-Albacete Martínez; Formal Analysis, Carlos Pérez-Albacete Martínez Investigation, Jose Luis Calvo-Guirado, José Eduardo Maté-Sánchez de Val; Resources, Sergio Gehrke; Data Curation, Sergio Gehrke; Writing-Original Draft Preparation, Jose Luis Calvo-Guirado; Writing-Review & Editing, Georgios E. Romanos, Rafael Arcesio Delgado-Ruiz; Visualization, Manuel Fernández-Domínguez; Supervision, Jose Luis Calvo-Guirado; Project Administration, Jose Luis Calvo-Guirado, Manuel Maiquez-Gosálvez; Funding Acquisition, Jose Luis Calvo-Guirado, Manuel Maiquez-Gosálvez".

Conflicts of Interest: The authors declare no conflict of interest.

References

1. Horowitz, R.; Holtzclaw, D.; Rosen, P.S. A review on alveolar ridge preservation following tooth extraction. *J. Evid. Based Dent. Pract.* **2012**, *12*, 149–160. [CrossRef]
2. Nanci, A. *Ten Cate's Oral Histology*, 7th ed.; Elsevier Inc.: Atlanta, GA, USA, 2008; pp. 202–211.
3. Min, B.M. *Oral Biochemistry*; Daehan Narae Pub Co.: Seoul, Korea, 2007; pp. 22–26.
4. Bhaskar, S.N. *Orban's Oral Histology and Embryology*, 9th ed.; Mosby Co.: Saint Louis, MO, USA, 1980.
5. Kim, Y.K.; Kim, S.G.; Byeon, J.H.; Lee, H.J.; Um, I.U.; Lim, S.C. Development of a novel bone grafting material using autogenous teeth. *Oral Surg. Oral Med. Oral Pathol. Oral Radiol. Endod.* **2010**, *109*, 496503. [CrossRef] [PubMed]
6. Murata, M.; Maki, F.; Sato, D.; Shibata, T.; Arisue, M. Bone augmentation by onlay implant using recombinant human BMP-2 and collagen on adult rat skull without periosteum. *Clin. Oral Impl. Res.* **2000**, *11*, 289–295. [CrossRef]
7. Murata, M.; Arisue, M.; Sato, D.; Sasaki, T.; Shibata, T.; Kuboki, Y. Bone induction in subcutaneous tissue in rats by a newly developed DNA-coated atelocollagen and bone morphogenetic protein. *Br. J. Oral Maxillofac. Surg.* **2002**, *40*, 131–135. [CrossRef] [PubMed]
8. Akazawa, T.; Murata, M.; Sasaki, T.; Tazaki, J.; Kobayashi, M.; Kanno, T.; Matsushima, K.; Arisue, M. Biodegradation and bioabsorption innovation of the functionally graded cattle-bone-originated apatite with blood compatibility. *J. Biomed. Mater. Res.* **2006**, *76*, 44–51. [CrossRef] [PubMed]
9. Murata, M.; Akazawa, T.; Tazaki, J.; Ito, K.; Sasaki, T.; Yamamoto, M.; Tabata, Y.; Arisue, M. Blood permeability of a novel ceramic scaffold for bone morphogenetic protein-2. *J. Biomed. Mater. Res.* **2007**, *81*, 469–475. [CrossRef] [PubMed]
10. Akazawa, T.; Murata, M.; Hino, J.; Nakamura, K.; Tazaki, J.; Kikuchi, M.; Arisue, M. Materials design and application of demineralized dentin/apatite composite granules derived from human teeth. *Arch. Bioceram. Res.* **2007**, *7*, 25–28.
11. Kim, S.G.; Kim, H.K.; Lim, S.C. Combined implantation of particulate dentin, plaster of Paris, and a bone xenograft (Bio-Oss) for bone regeneration in rats. *J. Craniomaxillofac. Surg.* **2001**, *29*, 282–288.
12. Kim, S.G.; Chung, C.H.; Kim, Y.K.; Park, J.C.; Lim, S.C. The use of particulate dentin–plaster of Paris combination with/without platelet-rich plasma in the treatment of bone defects around implants. *Int. J. Oral Maxillofac. Implants* **2002**, *17*, 86–94. [PubMed]
13. Kim, S.Y.; Kim, S.G.; Lim, S.C.; Bae, C.S. Effects on bone formation in ovariectomized rats after implantation of tooth ash and plaster of Paris mixture. *J. Oral Maxillofac. Surg.* **2004**, *62*, 852–857. [CrossRef] [PubMed]
14. Choi, D.K.; Kim, S.G.; Lim, S.C. The effect of particulate dentin–plaster of Paris combination with/without fibrin glue in the treatment of bone defects around implants. *Hosp. Dent.* **2007**, *19*, 121–126.
15. Kim, Y.K.; Yeo, H.H.; Ryu, C.H.; Lee, H.B.; Byun, U.R.; Cho, J.E. An experimental study on the tissue reaction of toothash implanted in mandible body of the mature dog. *J. Korean Assoc. Maxillofac. Plast. Reconstr. Surg.* **1993**, *15*, 129–136.

16. Kim, Y.K.; Yeo, H.H.; Cho, J.O. The experimental study of implantation combined with toothash and plaster of paris in the rats: Comparison according to the mixing ratio. *J. Korean Assoc. Maxillofac. Plast. Reconstr. Surg.* **1996**, *18*, 26–32.
17. Kim, Y.K.; Kim, S.G.; Yun, P.Y. Autogenous teeth used for bone grafting: A comparison with traditional grafting materials. *Oral Surg. Oral Med. Oral Pathol. Oral Radiol.* **2014**, *117*, e39–45. [CrossRef] [PubMed]
18. Kim, Y.-K.; Lee, J.; Um, I.-W.; Kim, K.-W.; Murata, M.; Akazawa, T.; Mitsugi, M. Tooth-derived bone graft material. *J. Korean Assoc. Oral Maxillofac. Surg.* **2013**, *39*, 103–111.
19. Andersson, L.; Blomlof, L.; Lindskog, S.; Feiglin, B.; Hammarstrom, L. Tooth ankylosis. Clinical, radiographic and histological assessments. *Int. J. Oral Surg.* **1984**, *13*, 423–431. [CrossRef]
20. Binderman, I.; Hallel, G.; Casp, N.; Yaffe, A. A Novel Procedure to Process Extracted Teeth for Immediate Grafting of Autogenous Dentin. *J. Interdiscipl. Med. Dent. Sci.* **2014**, *2*. [CrossRef]
21. Valdec, S.; Pasic, P.; Soltermann, A.; Thoma, D.; Stadlinger, B.; Rücker, M. Alveolar ridge preservation with autologous particulated dentin—A case series. *Int. J. Implant Dent.* **2017**, *3*, 12. [CrossRef] [PubMed]
22. Calvo Guirado, J.L. Nuevo procedimiento para procesar los dientes extraídos como injerto en alveolos postextracción. *Gaceta Dent.* **2017**, *290*, 96–113.
23. Malmgren, B. Ridge preservation/decoronation. *J. Endod.* **2013**, *39*, S67–S72. [CrossRef] [PubMed]
24. Park, C.H.; Abramson, Z.R.; Taba, M., Jr.; Jin, Q.; Chang, J.; Kreider, J.M.; Goldstein, S.A.; Giannobile, W.V. Three-dimensional micro-computed tomographic imaging of alveolar bone in experimental bone loss or repair. *J. Periodontol.* **2007**, *78*, 273–281. [CrossRef] [PubMed]
25. Yeomans, J.D.; Urist, M.R. Bone induction by decalcified implanted into oral, osseous and muscle tissues. *Arch. Oral Biol.* **1967**, *12*, 999–1008. [CrossRef]
26. Huggins, C.; Wiseman, S.; Reddi, A.H. Transformation of fibroblasts by allogeneic and xenogeneic transplants of demineralized tooth and bone. *J. Exp. Med.* **1970**, *132*, 1250–1258. [CrossRef] [PubMed]
27. Kim, Y.K.; Kim, S.G.; Yun, P.Y.; Yeo, I.S.; Jin, S.C.; Oh, J.S.; Kim, H.J.; Yu, S.K.; Lee, S.Y.; Kim, J.S.; Um, I.W.; Jeong, M.A.; et al. Autogenous teeth used for bone grafting: A comparison with traditional grafting materials. *Oral Surg. Oral Med. Oral Pathol. Oral Radiol.* **2014**, *117*, e39–e45. [CrossRef] [PubMed]
28. Andersson, L. Dentin xenografts to experimental bone defects in rabbit tibia are ankylosed and undergo osseous replacement. *Dent. Traumatol.* **2010**, *26*, 398–402. [CrossRef] [PubMed]
29. Kim, S.G.; Yeo, H.H.; Kim, Y.K. The clinical study of implantation of toothash combined with plaster of Paris: Long-term followup study. *J. Korean Assoc. Maxillofac. Plast. Reconstr. Surg.* **1996**, *18*, 771–777.
30. Kim, Y.K.; Yeo, H.H.; Park, I.S.; Cho, J.O. The experimental study on the healing process after the inlay implantation of toothash-plaster mixture block. *J. Korean Assoc. Maxillofac. Plast. Reconstr. Surg.* **1996**, *18*, 253–260.
31. Kim, Y.K. Bone graft material using teeth. *J. Korean Assoc. Oral Maxillofac. Surg.* **2012**, *38*, 134–138. [CrossRef]
32. Kim, Y.K. The experimental study of the implantation of toothash and plaster of Paris and guided tissue regeneration using Lyodura. *J. Korean Assoc. Oral Maxillofac. Surg.* **1996**, *22*, 297–306.
33. Pang, K.-M.; Um, I.-W.; Kim, Y.-K.; Woo, J.-M.; Kim, S.-M.; Lee, J.-H. Autogenous demineralized dentin matrix from extracted tooth for the augmentation of alveolar bone defect: A prospective randomized clinical trial in comparison with anorganic bovine bone. *Clin. Oral Implants Res.* **2017**, *28*, 809–815. [CrossRef] [PubMed]

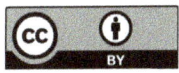

© 2018 by the authors. Licensee MDPI, Basel, Switzerland. This article is an open access article distributed under the terms and conditions of the Creative Commons Attribution (CC BY) license (http://creativecommons.org/licenses/by/4.0/).

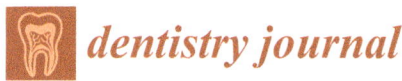

Article

Evaluation of an In Situ Hardening β-Tricalcium Phosphate Graft Material for Alveolar Ridge Preservation. A Histomorphometric Animal Study in Pigs

Minas Leventis [1,*], George Agrogiannis [2], Peter Fairbairn [3], Orestis Vasiliadis [1], Danai Papavasileiou [4], Evangelia Theodoropoulou [1], Robert Horowitz [5] and Demos Kalyvas [4]

1. Laboratory of Experimental Surgery and Surgical Research N. S. Christeas, Medical School, University of Athens, 75 M. Assias Street, 115 27 Athens, Greece; orestis@vasiliadis.net (O.V.); eva_theod@yahoo.gr (E.T.)
2. Department of Pathology, Medical School, University of Athens, 75 M. Assias Street, 115 27 Athens, Greece; agrojohn@med.uoa.gr
3. Department of Periodontology and Implant Dentistry, School of Dentistry, University of Detroit Mercy, 2700 Martin Luther King Jr Boulevard, Detroit, MI 48208, USA; peterdent66@aol.com
4. Department of Oral and Maxillofacial Surgery, Dental School, University of Athens, 2 Thivon Street, 115 27 Athens, Greece; d.pap.mes@gmail.com (D.P.); demkal@dent.uoa.gr (D.K.)
5. Departments of Periodontics, Implant Dentistry, and Oral Surgery, New York University College of Dentistry, 345 E 24th Street, New York, NY 10010, USA; rah7@nyu.edu
* Correspondence: mlevent@dent.uoa.gr; Tel.: +44-207-937-2160

Received: 21 April 2018; Accepted: 6 June 2018; Published: 2 July 2018

Abstract: The purpose of this study was to investigate the effectiveness of a resorbable alloplastic in situ hardening bone grafting material for alveolar ridge preservation in a swine model. Seven Landrace pigs were used. In each animal, the maxillary left and right deciduous second molars were extracted, and extraction sites were either grafted with a resorbable alloplastic in situ hardening bone substitute, composed of beta-tricalcium phosphate (β-TCP) granules coated with poly(lactic-co-glycolic) acid (PLGA), or left unfilled to heal spontaneously. Animals were euthanized after 12 weeks, and the bone tissue was analyzed histologically and histomorphometrically. Linear changes of ridge width were also clinically measured and analyzed. Pronounced bone regeneration was found in both experimental and control sites, with no statistically significant differences. At the experimental sites, most of the alloplastic grafting material was resorbed and remnants of the graft particles were severely decreased in size. Moreover, experimental sites showed, in a statistically nonsignificant way, less mean horizontal dimensional reduction of the alveolar ridge (7.69%) compared to the control sites (8.86%). In conclusion, the β-TCP/PLGA biomaterial performed well as a biocompatible resorbable in situ hardening bone substitute when placed in intact extraction sockets in this animal model.

Keywords: Alveolar ridge preservation; β-tricalcium phosphate; bone regeneration; bone substitutes; animal study

1. Introduction

Clinical trials and experimental preclinical studies have shown that the grafting of extraction sockets constitutes a predictable and reliable way to preserve the dimensions and architecture of the alveolar ridge [1–6]. Such measures involve the use of different kinds of bone grafts, barrier membranes and growth-factor preparations, and many different surgical techniques and protocols have been proposed [7–10]. Currently, it is still unclear which material or surgical method is the most effective in limiting post-extraction resorption while assisting in regenerating adequate vital bone. According to Yip et al. [11], the ideal bone grafting material should have specific attributes. It should be osteoconductive, osteoinductive and biocompatible. It is important to be gradually replaced by newly formed bone, exhibiting controlled breakdown and resorption, and it should be able to maintain the ridge contour in the augmented site. Moreover, it should have satisfactory mechanical properties and no risk of disease transmission.

In contemporary oral and implant surgery, bone substitutes are widely researched and utilized as an alternative to autogenous bone, in an attempt to avoid complicated procedures and reduce treatment time [12]. Alloplasts represent a group of synthetic and highly biocompatible bone grafting materials [13]. The use of alloplastic biomaterials does not pose a risk of transmitting infections or diseases, and their availability is unlimited [14–16]. Calcium phosphate ceramics are bioactive osteoconductive materials, and there is strong experimental evidence that they also have osteoinductive properties, while promoting neovascularization [17–21]. Among ceramics, beta-tricalcium phosphate (β-TCP) is widely used in orthopedics and in dentistry, mostly in the form of particulate grafts or cements. In order to improve its biological performance and mechanical properties, β-TCP can be combined with other synthetic materials [15,22–29]. Coating the β-TCP granules with poly(lactic-*co*-glycolic) acid (PLGA) produces an in situ hardening, stable, porous biomaterial that serves as a bioactive scaffold for bone reconstruction, while reducing the need for additional membranes to retain and stabilize the graft material in the bone defect [24,25,27].

Moreover, the increased stability throughout the grafted site, and the reduced micromotions of the graft particles might lead to enhanced bone regeneration. Such micromovements between bone and any implanted material may trigger differentiation of mesenchymal cells to fibroblasts instead of osteoblasts, and inhibit bone formation, resulting in the development of fibrous tissue [30–32].

The aim of this experimental study was to test the hypothesis that filling intact extraction sockets with a resorbable alloplastic in situ hardening biomaterial, consisting of β-TCP and PLGA, will limit resorption of the alveolar ridge, and assist in regeneration of new bone, compared to sites subjected to spontaneous healing, in a swine model.

2. Materials and Methods

2.1. Surgical Procedures

Seven 4-month-old female Landrace pigs, each weighing 18 kg ($\pm$2 kg), were used in this study with the approval of the Institutional Animal Care and Use Committee of the Veterinary Department, Greek Ministry of Rural Development and Veterinary, Attica Prefecture, Greece (8042/10-12-1014). The animals were allowed 7 days from their arrival to the N.S. Christeas animal research facility of the University of Athens Medical School, Athens, Greece to acclimatize to their new environment. Before and after operation were fed a balanced soft diet and water *ad libitum*, and caged individually in a standard manner.

Animals were sedated with an intramuscular injection of 2 mg/kg body weight xylazine (Rompun, Bayer Hellas AG, Athens, Greece) plus 25 mg/kg body weight ketamine (Imalgene, Merial, Lyon, France). In each animal, the left and right second deciduous molars of the maxilla were "atraumatically" extracted without raising a flap (Figure 1, Video S1).

Intraoral local infiltrations with articaine and adrenaline 1:20,000 were performed buccally and palatally for hemostasis. Teeth were sectioned with a Lindemann bur under copious irrigation with sterile saline, each root was independently mobilized with periotomes, and removed with forceps, in order not to damage the surrounding soft and hard tissues, especially in the buccal aspect. Subsequently, the developing bud of the underlying second premolar, located at the apical part of the socket, was removed using a sharp Lucas bone curette. All sites were thoroughly debrided from soft tissues, and rinsed with sterile saline. The buccal bone plate in all cases had to be intact (4-wall extraction sockets).

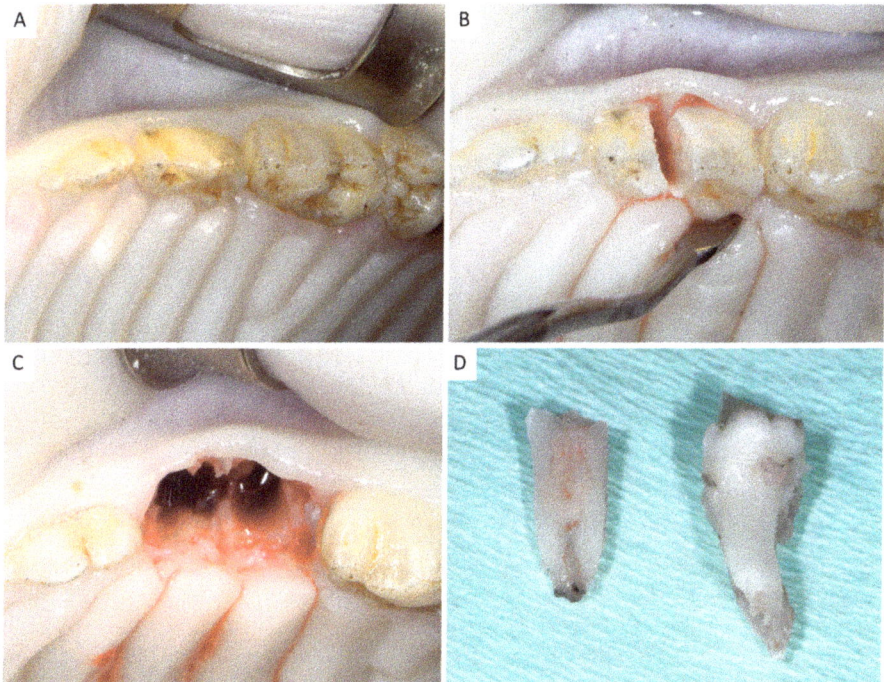

Figure 1. (**A**) Initial clinical view; (**B**) The deciduous maxillary second molar was sectioned, and each root was separately mobilized and extracted; (**C**) Clinical view of the site immediately after extraction; (**D**) The extracted tooth.

The extraction sites were either grafted (experimental sites, $n = 10$) or left unfilled (control sites, $n = 4$). A randomization technique using cards was followed. Paper cards were consecutively marked as "experiment" ($n = 10$) or "control" ($n = 4$). All cards were enclosed in identical sealed envelopes. Upon completion of each extraction, a clinical assistant not involved in the study was asked to open an envelope. A resorbable alloplastic in situ hardening bone grafting material (GUIDOR *easy-graft* CLASSIC, Sunstar Suisse SA, Etoy, Switzerland) was utilized to fill the experimental sites. This bone substitute is composed of β-TCP granules coated with a thin (10 μm) layer of PLGA. The biomaterial is preloaded in a sterile plastic syringe (Figure 2A), and a liquid Biolinker^{TM} (*N*-methyl-2-pyrrolidone solution) is mixed in the syringe with the graft granules prior to injecting the material into the socket. The Biolinker^{TM} turns the coated granules into a sticky mass, and allows moldability of the biomaterial, which begins to progressively harden in situ after application in the socket and upon contact with blood [28]. The graft granules were condensed in order to occupy the whole volume of the socket up to the level of the surrounding host bone (Figure 2B, Video S2), and the sites were closed in a tension-free manner with interrupted resorbable 3-0 sutures (Vicryl, Ethicon, Johnson & Johnson, Somerville, NJ, USA) (Figure 2C).

Each animal received intramuscularly antibiotics (enrofloxacin, Baytril 5%, Bayer Hellas AG, Athens, Greece) and analgesics (carpofen, Rimadyl, Pfizer Hellas SA, Athens, Greece) for 3 days postoperatively.

All animals were euthanized 12 weeks postoperatively with an intravenous injection of 100 mg/kg sodium thiopental (Pentothal, Abbott Hellas, Athens, Greece), and the parts of the jaws including the healed extraction sockets were surgically harvested.

At baseline and at 12 weeks, the width of the ridge was directly measured using a caliper 3 mm below the central part of the crest.

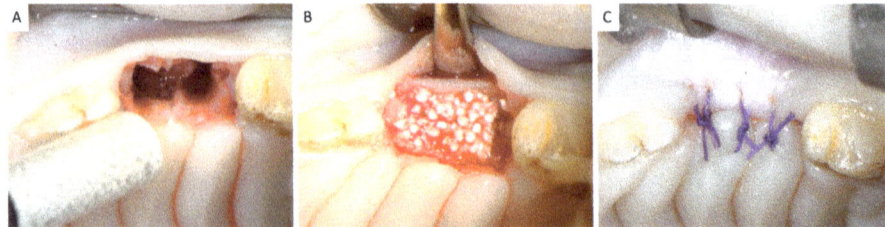

Figure 2. (**A**,**B**) The experimental sites were grafted with the resorbable alloplastic in situ hardening bone substitute; (**C**) All sites were closed without tension.

2.2. Histological and Histomorphometric Evaluation

The block specimens were fixed in 10% formalin for 2 days, and subsequently decalcified in bone decalcification solution (Diapath S.p.a., Martinengo, Italy) for 14 days. After routine processing, slices were obtained from the central part of the specimens using a saw (Exakt saw 312, Exakt Apparatebau GmbH, Norderstedt, Germany), embedded in paraffin, sectioned longitudinally into multiple 3 μm-thick sections, and stained with hematoxylin and eosin (H&E). For qualitative and morphologic analysis of the remodeling process, the stained preparations were examined under a light microscope (Nikon Eclipse 80, Nikon, Tokyo, Japan) at a minimum 20× magnification, and the entire section was evaluated. For histomorphometric analysis, images of each section were acquired with a digital camera microscope unit (Nikon DS-2MW, Nikon, Tokyo, Japan), and used to trace the areas identified as old maxillary bone, newly formed bone, residual graft, and connective tissue. A combination of Adobe PhotoShop (Adobe Systems Inc., San Jose, CA, USA) and image analysis software (Image-Pro Plus v. 5.1, Media Cybernetics, Rockville, MD, USA) was used to create individual layers of newly formed bone, biomaterial particles, and connective tissue. For each site, the following parameters were assessed: % new bone, % residual graft, % connective tissue, presence of inflammation, and complications. A single observer blinded to the clinical data carried out all analyses and measurements.

2.3. Statistical Analysis

Statistical analysis was performed using SPSS software (v. 17, SPSS Inc., Chicago, IL, USA). Data were expressed as mean ± standard deviation (SD). The Kolmogorov–Smirnov test was used for normality analysis of the parameters. A comparison of variables between the two groups was performed using the independent samples *t*-test or Mann–Whitney test in case of violation of normality. Two-factor mixed factorial ANOVA was used to examine the interaction between the socket treatment factor and the time factor. Paired samples *t*-test was used for comparison of different time measurements of ridge width for each group. Comparison of percentage change of ridge width from initial evaluation to 12 weeks postoperative between the two groups was analyzed using the independent samples *t*-test or Mann–Whitney test in case of violation of normality. Using the analysis of covariance model (ANCOVA), the absolute change from initial assessment to 12 weeks postoperative of ridge width variable between the two groups was compared. All tests were two-sided, and statistical significance was set at $p < 0.05$.

3. Results

3.1. Overall

The postoperative course of all animals was uneventful. At 12 weeks, all sites were completely healed, covered by keratinized soft tissues (Figure 3). There were no clinical signs of local inflammation or infection.

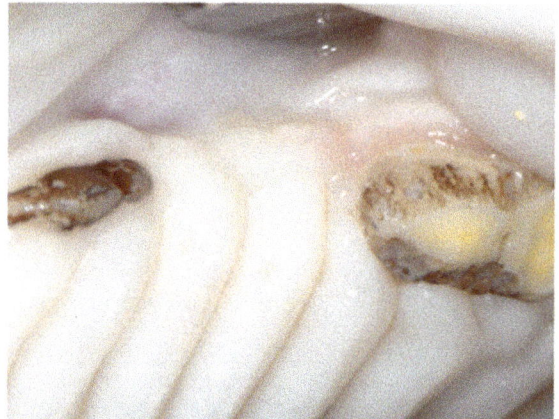

Figure 3. Normal healing after 12 weeks.

3.2. Alveolar Ridge Dimensional Changes

After 12 weeks, all sites underwent several degrees of atrophy. The ridge width changed during the observation period in the same way for both groups (Table 1). Experimental extraction sites grafted with the alloplastic bone substitute showed less mean horizontal dimensional reduction of the alveolar ridge compared to sites subjected to spontaneous healing. However, this difference was not statistically significant (Table 2).

Table 1. Comparison of absolute values of alveolar ridge width between groups at each time point.

	N	Mean (mm)	SD	*p*-Value
Initial				
Graft	10	7.93	0.44	0.319
Control	4	7.63	0.63	
12 weeks postop				
Graft	10	7.32	0.59	0.233
Control	4	6.93	0.29	

Table 2. Evaluation of percentage change of ridge width from initial to 12 weeks postoperative for experimental and control sites.

	N	Mean (%)	SD	*p*-Value
Initial to 12 weeks postop				
Graft	10	−7.69	5.46	0.727
Control	4	−8.86	5.92	

3.3. Histology

At 12 weeks, both experimental and control sites were filled with regenerated bone, bone marrow and connective tissue. At the periphery of all sockets, native cortical bone could be identified in continuity with the newly formed cancellous bone in the center. The entrances of the sockets were sealed with woven bone of immature state, which was covered by newly formed periosteum-like connective tissue with a linear arrangement of osteoblasts. Histologically, no soft tissue ingrowth was observed. All sockets were covered by regular stratified squamous keratinized epithelium. At the experimental sites, most of the alloplastic grafting material particles were resorbed, and the remnants were severely decreased in size (Figure 4).

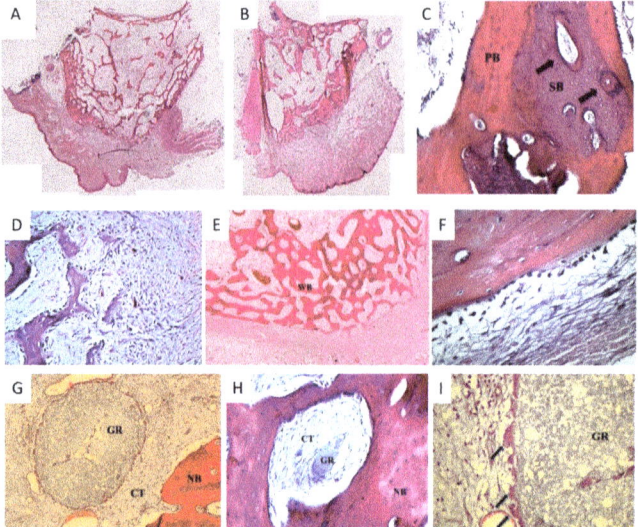

Figure 4. Representative histological pictures (H&E staining). (**A**) Site grafted with the resorbable alloplastic biomaterial at 12 weeks. The site is filled with regenerated bone, bone marrow and connective tissue. At the periphery of the socket, native cortical bone can be identified in continuity with the newly formed cancellous bone in the center. At this time point, most of the *easy-graft* CLASSIC particles have been resorbed; (**B**) Nongrafted extraction site at 12 weeks. Regenerated bone showing active remodeling; (**C**) At the center, mature secondary bone (SB) with harversian systems (arrows) can be observed, surrounded by less mature primary lamellar bone (PB). These types of bone are clearly separated by cement or reversal lines; (**D**) Newly formed bone trabeculae with osteoblast lining at the periphery, and connective tissue with numerous mesenchymal cells; (**E**) Newly formed woven bone (WB) sealing the entrance of the extraction socket; (**F**) Periosteum-like connective tissue covering the periphery of the socket with linear arrangement of osteoblasts; (**G**) Residual granule of *easy-graft* CLASSIC (GR) surrounded by connective tissue (CT) and newly formed bone (NB); (**H**) Remnant of *easy-graft* CLASSIC (GR) surrounded by a few multinucleated cells and connective tissue (CT) with blood vessels, fibroblasts, and collagen fibers. At the periphery, newly formed bone (NB) is present; (**I**) Multinuclear cells (arrows) lining the periphery of a granule of *easy-graft* CLASSIC (GR).

3.4. Histomorphometry

The results of the histomorphometric analysis are shown in Table 3. At 12 weeks, more new bone formation was observed in sockets grafted with *easy-graft* CLASSIC compared to the sites that healed spontaneously. However, a statistically significant difference regarding osteogenesis was not demonstrated between the two groups. Experimental grafted sites exhibited small amounts of residual biomaterial at this time point.

Table 3. Percentages of new bone, connective tissue and residual graft occupying the sockets.

Parameter	Group	N	Mean	SD	p-Value
New bone %	Graft	10	20.33	8.10	0.268
	Control	4	15.40	3.01	
Connective tissue %	Graft	10	76.24	10.01	0.198
	Control	4	83.26	1.63	
Residual graft %	Graft	10	0.26	0.38	-
	Control	4	-	-	

4. Discussion

In this animal study, we investigated the effects of filling extraction sites in a swine model with a resorbable alloplastic in situ hardening bone grafting material.

After a 12-week healing period, all experimental sites healed uneventfully, with no clinical signs of local complications or infection. Histologically, the absence of acute inflammatory infiltrates and foreign body reactions confirms the good biocompatibility of the alloplastic biomaterial used.

The histologic and histomorphometric results showed pronounced new bone formation in both groups. Experimental sites, where ridge preservation measures were applied, showed more newly formed bone volume compared to the empty unassisted sites where natural healing occurred. However, our findings were not statistically significant. According to the current relevant literature, conflicting evidence exists on the benefit of alveolar ridge preservation techniques at the histologic level. Such techniques with the use of grafting materials do not appear to promote *de novo* hard tissue formation routinely. In addition, some graft materials may interfere with healing [1,3]. Grafting has been reported to impede the healing process in the fresh extraction socket model [31]. Biomaterials in a well-maintained space like the intact socket may arrest or delay bone formation, as it is reported that bone substitutes may modify the normal healing process and inhibit bone formation in grafted sockets compared to nongrafted sites [33–35].

In accordance with the present study's observations, Leventis et al. [24], in a case series clinical study analyzing bone biopsies of human extraction sockets grafted with *easy-graft* CLASSIC, reported that after 4 months of healing, newly formed bone occupied 24.4% of the regenerated sites. These findings are similar to the results of the present study, where 20.33% of newly formed bone was observed at the animal extraction sockets at 12 weeks.

When regenerating alveolar bone, with the use of bone substitutes, the grafting material must have an appropriate resorption time in relation to new bone formation. It is also important to be replaced by host bone [11,36]. The long-term presence of residual nonresorbable or slowly resorbable particles of the graft might interfere with the bone healing mechanism and the remodeling of the new tissue, having a negative effect on the overall quality and architecture of the reconstructed bone. This is of great importance if the placement of a dental implant is planned, as bone-to-implant contact, initial implant stability and long-term function might be impaired in the presence of a high volume of nonresorbable graft particles in the regenerated bone tissue [36]. In the present study, the material used exhibited pronounced resorption after 12 weeks, being almost completely resorbed (0.26% of the tissue volume). Multinucleated giant cells were observed that seemed to be actively phagocytizing dissolved or partially dissolved graft granules. These findings confirm earlier animal studies showing fast resorption of β-TCP with time, and imply that the breakdown of β-TCP seems to be a combination of dissolution and direct cell-mediated resorption [34,37,38]. However, human extraction sockets grafted with *easy-graft* CLASSIC showed 12.9% residual biomaterial after 12 weeks [24].

The fast resorption of *easy-graft* CLASSIC shown in the present study can be explained by the fact that the material was placed into intact four-wall sockets, meaning that the high vascularity from the surrounding thick bone plates might have resulted in pronounced resorption by multinucleated phagocytes derived from the host blood. The findings could also be explained by the higher metabolic activity of the animal model used in the present study. Finally, these findings of pronounced graft resorption could be attributed to washout of some material from the grafted socket during healing due to friction induced by mastication of the pig. However, the biomechanical in situ hardening characteristics of *easy-graft* CLASSIC provide adequate stability to the material as the granules adhere to each other. In this respect, they form a hard scaffold that interlocks into the defect, and therefore it can be left uncovered to heal by secondary intention. Data from human clinical studies and case reports show that the self-hardening characteristics of such alloplastic grafting materials facilitate the secondary healing of grafted sockets, without evidence of washout of the uncovered biomaterial in the oral environment [24,26,39]. Moreover, in the present study, the grafted sites were sutured tension-free, so no material was exposed postoperatively. However, in contrast to human studies, in this experimental animal model, it was not possible to monitor and observe clinically any wound dehiscence and/or washout of grafting material during the healing period. Clinical observations were possible only on the day of surgery and the day of euthanasia. In order to clinically evaluate the extraction sites at any other time point in between, strong medical sedation of the animals would be necessary, which could threaten their health.

Tooth extraction not only results in resorption of the alveolar bone, but also triggers a structural change in the overlying soft tissue [40]. Human studies reporting data on horizontal hard and soft tissue changes have shown a reduction of 0.1–3.8 mm, with a weighted mean reduction of 1.3 mm, after extraction without applying any grafting procedures [40]. Recent systematic reviews have demonstrated that alveolar ridge preservation techniques may contribute to less ridge width reduction than what occurs following natural socket healing, although such techniques do not totally eliminate post-extraction resorption [1–4].

In this study, we measured in each group the combined hard and soft tissue change in the horizontal dimension, following extraction, in order to evaluate the alterations of overall ridge width. Comparing the absolute change of the horizontal dimension from baseline to 12 weeks postoperatively between the two groups, the present results showed that the experimental grafted sites underwent less resorption than the control nongrafted sites. However, the differences between the two groups were not statistically significant. It is important that in the present study, similar to other studies [40], the overall dimensions of the alveolar ridge were analyzed corresponding to alterations of the soft and hard tissues. It is stated that the soft tissue may increase in dimension to partially compensate for the resorption of the hard tissue. For this reason, such assessments may not be appropriate to evaluate the effectiveness of ridge preservation procedures regarding the alveolar bone [4,41]. In the present study, only linear measurements of the width of the ridge were made. Volumetric measurements of the buccal and occlusal volumes would provide more accurate data regarding the loss of volume and changes of the ridge profile in both groups.

The statistically nonsignificant results in the present study may be attributed to several reasons. A larger sample could have resulted in statistically significant results; however, for ethical reasons and to comply with the guidelines of the ethical committee, the smallest number of animals was used in the study. Another explanation could be the minimally invasive surgical technique utilized and the use of four-wall sockets with an intact thick buccal bone. An important factor determining the quality of the socket after extraction is the presence of the buccal wall, meaning that these sites have high regenerative potential and show less resorption even following natural spontaneous healing without the aid of Guided Bone Regeneration measures [42]. In contrast, sockets with thin (1 mm or less) or defective fenestrated buccal walls are prone to more atrophy, up to 56% of horizontal resorption [43,44]. A thin cortical buccal plate has poor vascularity, and contains few marrow spaces. So, after extraction and especially when a buccal full-thickness flap is raised, which would compromise the blood supply from the periosteum more, it will resorb quickly, resulting in pronounced atrophy of the site. As shown in a different experimental study, it can be postulated that the effect of grafting the extraction sites with *easy-graft* would be more pronounced if sockets with thin, defective, or missing buccal plates were treated [45]. It is reasonable that in such defective sites, where more pronounced atrophy is expected after spontaneous natural healing, the above grafting measures may have a greater impact on preserving the width of the ridge, and the possible differences between the experimental and control groups might be more significant and conclusive.

5. Conclusions

Within the limits of the present experimental study, it can be concluded that the resorbable alloplastic bone substitute showed excellent biocompatibility and can support new bone formation when placed in intact extraction sockets for alveolar ridge preservation in this animal model. The use of *easy-graft* CLASSIC did not impede the healing of fresh four-wall extraction sites, as reported for other bone graft substitutes, while the in situ hardening characteristics of the material can improve the handling and stability of the sites, allowing for minimally invasive procedures.

Supplementary Materials: The following are available online at http://www.mdpi.com/2304-6767/6/3/27/s1: Video S1: Minimally invasive extraction of the deciduous maxillary second molar. Video S2: Grafting of the extraction site (experimental group) with the in situ hardening alloplastic biomaterial.

Author Contributions: All of the named authors were involved in the work leading to publication of this paper and read the paper before this submission. M.L., P.F., O.V., E.T. and D.P. performed the whole in vivo experiment; G.A. made the histological slides and performed the histological analysis; and M.L., P.F., R.H. and D.K. designed the experiment and gave final approval of the version to be published with full management of this manuscript.

Acknowledgments: The authors would like to acknowledge Antonis Galanos, BSc, PhD, for his support in the statistical analysis of the data, and the animal care team at the Laboratory of Experimental Surgery and Surgical Research, N.S. Christeas, Athens, Greece, for assistance during surgery.

Conflicts of Interest: The authors declare no conflict of interest.

References

1. Jambhekar, S.; Kernen, F.; Bidra, A.S. Clinical and histologic outcomes of socket grafting after flapless tooth extraction: A systematic review of randomized controlled clinical trials. *J. Prosthet. Dent.* **2015**, *113*, 371–382. [CrossRef] [PubMed]
2. Vittorini Orgeas, G.; Clementini, M.; De Risi, V.; De Sanctis, M. Surgical techniques for alveolar socket preservation: A systematic review. *Int. J. Oral Maxillofac. Implants* **2013**, *28*, 1049–1061. [CrossRef] [PubMed]
3. Horváth, A.; Mardas, N.; Mezzomo, L.A.; Needleman, I.G.; Donos, N. Alveolar ridge preservation. A systematic review. *Clin. Oral Investig.* **2013**, *17*, 341–363. [CrossRef] [PubMed]
4. Wang, R.E.; Lang, N.P. Ridge preservation after tooth extraction. *Clin. Oral Implants Res.* **2012**, *23* (Suppl. 6), 147–156. [CrossRef] [PubMed]
5. Fickl, S.; Zuhr, O.; Wachtel, H.; Bolz, W.; Huerzeler, M.B. Hard tissue alterations after socket preservation: An experimental study in the beagle dog. *Clin. Oral Implants Res.* **2008**, *19*, 1111–1118. [CrossRef] [PubMed]
6. Keith, J.D., Jr.; Salama, M.A. Ridge preservation and augmentation using regenerative materials to enhance implant predictability and esthetics. *Compend. Contin. Educ. Dent.* **2007**, *28*, 614–621. [PubMed]
7. Horowitz, R.; Holtzclaw, D.; Rosen, P.S. A review on alveolar ridge preservation following tooth extraction. *J. Evid. Based Dent. Pract.* **2012**, *12* (Suppl. 3), 149–160. [CrossRef]
8. Horowitz, R.A.; Leventis, M.D.; Rohrer, M.D.; Prasad, H.S. Bone grafting: History, rationale, and selection of materials and techniques. *Compend. Contin. Educ. Dent.* **2014**, *35* (Suppl. 4), 1–6. [PubMed]
9. Collins, J.R.; Jiménez, E.; Martínez, C.; Polanco, R.T.; Hirata, R.; Mousa, R.; Coelho, P.G.; Bonfante, E.A.; Tovar, N. Clinical and histological evaluation of socket grafting using different types of bone substitute in adult patients. *Implant Dent.* **2014**, *23*, 489–495. [CrossRef] [PubMed]
10. Barallat, L.; Ruiz-Magaz, V.; Levi, P.A., Jr.; Mareque-Bueno, S.; Galindo-Moreno, P.; Nart, J. Histomorphometric results in ridge preservation procedures comparing various graft materials in extraction sockets with nongrafted sockets in humans: A systematic review. *Implant Dent.* **2014**, *23*, 539–554. [CrossRef] [PubMed]
11. Yip, I.; Ma, L.; Mattheos, N.; Dard, M.; Lang, N.P. Defect healing with various bone substitutes. *Clin. Oral Implants Res.* **2015**, *26*, 606–614. [CrossRef] [PubMed]
12. Valkova, V.; Ubaidha Maheen, C.; Pommer, B.; Rausch-Fan, X.; Seeman, R. Hot Topics in Clinical Oral Implants Research: Recent Trends in Literature Coverage. *Dent. J.* **2016**, *4*, E13. [CrossRef] [PubMed]
13. Gao, C.; Peng, S.; Feng, P.; Shuai, C. Bone biomaterials and interactions with stem cells. *Bone Res.* **2017**, *5*, 17059. [CrossRef] [PubMed]
14. Araújo, M.G.; Liljenberg, B.; Lindhe, J. β-tricalcium phosphate in the early phase of socket healing: An experimental study in the dog. *Clin. Oral Implants Res.* **2010**, *21*, 445–454. [CrossRef] [PubMed]
15. Harel, N.; Moses, O.; Palti, A.; Ormianer, Z. Long-term results of implants immediately placed into extraction sockets grafted with β-tricalcium phosphate: A retrospective study. *J. Oral Maxillofac. Surg.* **2013**, *71*, E63–E68. [CrossRef] [PubMed]
16. Trisi, P.; Rao, W.; Rebaudi, A.; Fiore, P. Histologic effect of pure-phase beta-tricalcium phosphate on bone regeneration in human artificial jawbone defects. *Int. J. Periodontics Restor. Dent.* **2003**, *23*, 69–78.

17. Henkel, J.; Woodruff, M.A.; Epari, D.R.; Steck, R.; Glatt, V.; Dickinson, I.C.; Choong, P.F.; Schuetz, M.A.; Hutmacher, D.W. Bone regeneration based on tissue engineering conceptions—A 21st century perspective. *Bone Res.* **2013**, *1*, 216–248. [CrossRef] [PubMed]
18. Yuan, H.; Fernandes, H.; Habibovic, P.; de Boer, J.; Barradas, A.M.; de Ruiter, A.; Walsh, W.R.; van Blitterswijk, C.A.; de Bruijn, J.D. Osteoinductive ceramics as a synthetic alternative to autologous bone grafting. *Proc. Nat. Acad. Sci. USA* **2010**, *107*, 13614–13619. [CrossRef] [PubMed]
19. Miron, R.J.; Zhang, Q.; Sculean, A.; Buser, D.; Pippenger, B.E.; Dard, M.; Shirakata, Y.; Chandad, F.; Zhang, Y. Osteoinductive potential of 4 commonly employed bone grafts. *Clin. Oral Investig.* **2016**, *20*, 2259–2265. [CrossRef] [PubMed]
20. Barradas, A.M.; Yuan, H.; van Blitterswijk, C.; Habibovic, P. Osteoinductive biomaterials: Current knowledge of properties, experimental models and biological mechanisms. *Eur. Cell. Mater.* **2010**, *21*, 407–429. [CrossRef]
21. Malhotra, A.; Habibovic, P. Calcium phosphates and angiogenesis: Implications and advances for bone regeneration. *Trends Biotechnol.* **2016**, *34*, 983–992. [CrossRef] [PubMed]
22. Palti, A.; Hoch, T. A concept for the treatment of various dental bone defects. *Implant Dent.* **2002**, *11*, 73–78. [CrossRef] [PubMed]
23. Fairbairn, P.; Leventis, M. Protocol for Bone Augmentation with Simultaneous Early Implant Placement: A Retrospective Multicenter Clinical Study. *Int. J. Dent.* **2015**, *2015*, 589135. [CrossRef] [PubMed]
24. Leventis, M.D.; Fairbairn, P.; Kakar, A.; Leventis, A.D.; Margaritis, V.; Lückerath, W.; Horowitz, R.A.; Rao, B.H.; Lindner, A.; Nagursky, H. Minimally invasive alveolar ridge preservation utilizing an in situ hardening β-tricalcium phosphate bone substitute: A multicenter case series. *Int. J. Dent.* **2016**, *2016*, 5406736. [CrossRef] [PubMed]
25. Schmidlin, P.R.; Nicholls, F.; Kruse, A.; Zwahlen, R.A.; Weber, F.E. Evaluation of moldable, in situ hardening calcium phosphate bone graft substitutes. *Clin. Oral Implants Res.* **2013**, *24*, 149–157. [CrossRef] [PubMed]
26. Khan, R.; Witek, L.; Breit, M.; Colon, D.; Tovar, N.; Janal, M.N.; Jimbo, R.; Coelho, P.G. Bone regenerative potential of modified biphasic graft materials. *Implant Dent.* **2015**, *24*, 149–154. [CrossRef] [PubMed]
27. Kakar, A.; Rao, B.H.S.; Hegde, S.; Deshpande, N.; Lindner, A.; Nagursky, H.; Patney, A.; Mahajan, H. Ridge preservation using an in situ hardening biphasic calcium phosphate (β-TCP/HA) bone graft substitute—A clinical, radiological, and histological study. *Int. J. Implant Dent.* **2017**, *3*, 25. [CrossRef] [PubMed]
28. Ruffieux, K. New syringe-delivered, moldable, alloplastic bone graft substitute. *Compend. Contin. Educ. Dent.* **2014**, *35* (Suppl. 4), 8–10. [PubMed]
29. Murray, K.A.; Collins, M.N.; O'Sullivan, R.P.; Ren, G.; Devine, D.M.; Murphy, A.; Sadło, J.; O'Sullivan, C.; McEvoy, B.; Vrain, O.; et al. Influence of gamma and electron beam sterilization on the stability of a premixed injectable calcium phosphate cement for trauma indications. *J. Mech. Behav. Biomed. Mater.* **2018**, *77*, 116–124. [CrossRef] [PubMed]
30. Dimitriou, R.; Mataliotakis, G.I.; Calori, G.M.; Giannoudis, P.V. The role of barrier membranes for guided bone regeneration and restoration of large bone defects: Current experimental and clinical evidence. *BMC Med.* **2012**, *10*, 81. [CrossRef] [PubMed]
31. Giannoudis, P.V.; Einhorn, T.A.; Marsh, D. Fracture healing: The diamond concept. *Injury* **2007**, *38*, S3–S6. [CrossRef]
32. Troedhan, A.; Schlichting, I.; Kurrek, A.; Wainwright, M. Primary implant stability in augmented sinuslift-sites after completed bone regeneration: A randomized controlled clinical study comparing four subantrally inserted biomaterials. *Sci. Rep.* **2014**, *4*, 5877. [CrossRef] [PubMed]
33. Carmagnola, D.; Adriaens, P.; Berglundh, T. Healing of human extraction sockets filled with Bio-Oss. *Clin. Oral Implants Res.* **2003**, *14*, 137–143. [CrossRef] [PubMed]
34. Hong, J.Y.; Lee, J.S.; Pang, E.K.; Jung, U.W.; Choi, S.H.; Kim, C.K. Impact of different synthetic bone fillers on healing of extraction sockets: An experimental study in dogs. *Clin. Oral Implants Res.* **2014**, *25*, E30–E37. [CrossRef] [PubMed]
35. Araújo, M.G.; Lindhe, J. Ridge preservation with the use of Bio-Oss collagen: A 6-month study in the dog. *Clin. Oral Implants Res.* **2009**, *20*, 433–440. [CrossRef] [PubMed]
36. Chan, H.L.; Lin, G.H.; Fu, J.H.; Wang, H.L. Alterations in bone quality after socket preservation with grafting materials: A systematic review. *Int. J. Oral Maxillofac. Implants* **2013**, *28*, 710–720. [CrossRef] [PubMed]

37. Artzi, Z.; Weinreb, M.; Givol, N.; Rohrer, M.D.; Nemcovsky, C.E.; Prasad, H.S.; Tal, H. Biomaterial Resorption Rate and Healing Site Morphology of Inorganic Bovine Bone and β-Tricalcium Phosphate in the Canine: A 24-month Longitudinal Histologic Study and Morphometric Analysis. *Int. J. Oral Maxillofac. Implants* **2004**, *19*, 357–368. [PubMed]
38. Jensen, S.S.; Broggini, N.; Hjørting-Hansen, E.; Schenk, R.; Buser, D. Bone healing and graft resorption of autograft, anorganic bovine bone and beta-tricalcium phosphate. A histologic and histomorphometric study in the mandibles of minipigs. *Clin. Oral Implants Res.* **2006**, *17*, 237–243. [CrossRef] [PubMed]
39. Leventis, M.D.; Fairbairn, P.; Horowitz, R.A. Extraction site preservation using an in-situ hardening alloplastic bone graft substitute. *Compend. Contin. Educ. Dent.* **2014**, *35* (Suppl. 4), 11–13. [PubMed]
40. Schropp, L.; Wenzel, A.; Kostopoulos, L.; Karring, T. Bone healing and soft tissue contour changes following single-tooth extraction: A clinical and radiographic 12-month prospective study. *Int. J. Periodontics Restor. Dent.* **2003**, *23*, 313–323.
41. Tan, W.L.; Wong, T.L.; Wong, M.C.; Lang, N.P. A systematic review of post-extractional alveolar hard and soft tissue dimensional changes in humans. *Clin. Oral Implants Res.* **2012**, *23* (Suppl. 5), 1–21. [CrossRef] [PubMed]
42. Elian, N.; Cho, S.C.; Froum, S.; Smith, R.B.; Tarnow, D.P. A simplified socket classification and repair technique. *Pract. Proced. Aesthet. Dent.* **2007**, *19*, 99–104. [PubMed]
43. Huynh-Ba, G.; Pjetursson, B.E.; Sanz, M.; Cecchinato, D.; Ferrus, J.; Lindhe, J.; Lang, N.P. Analysis of the socket bone wall dimensions in the upper maxilla in relation to immediate implant placement. *Clin Oral Implants Res.* **2010**, *21*, 37–42. [CrossRef] [PubMed]
44. Tarnow, D.P.; Chu, S.J. Human histologic verification of osseointegration of an immediate implant placed into a fresh extraction socket with excessive gap distance without primary flap closure, graft, or membrane: A case report. *Int. J. Periodontics Restor. Dent.* **2011**, *31*, 515–521.
45. Naenni, N.; Sapata, V.; Bienz, S.P.; Leventis, M.; Jung, R.; Hämmerle, C.H.; Thoma, D.S. Effect of flapless ridge preservation with two different alloplastic materials in sockets with buccal dehiscence defects—Volumetric and linear changes. *Clin. Oral Investig.* **2017**, *22*, 2187–2197. [CrossRef] [PubMed]

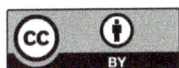

© 2018 by the authors. Licensee MDPI, Basel, Switzerland. This article is an open access article distributed under the terms and conditions of the Creative Commons Attribution (CC BY) license (http://creativecommons.org/licenses/by/4.0/).

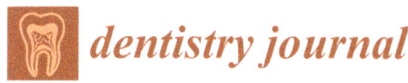

Review

Videoscope-Assisted Minimally Invasive Surgery (VMIS) for Bone Regeneration around Teeth and Implants: A Literature Review and Technique Update

Stephen K. Harrel

Department of Periodontology, Texas A&M College of Dentistry, Dallas, TX 75246, USA; skharrel@gmail.com; Tel.: +1-214-352-5304

Received: 14 June 2018; Accepted: 3 July 2018; Published: 6 July 2018

Abstract: Background—The literature related to minimally invasive periodontal surgery is reviewed. This includes the original minimally invasive surgery (MIS) procedure for bone regeneration, the modification of MIS for the minimally invasive surgery technique (MIST) and modified MIST (M-MIST) procedures, and the introduction of the videoscope for oral surgical procedures and the ability to perform videoscope-assisted minimally invasive surgery (VMIS). The evolution from MIS through MIST to the current VMIS is reviewed. The results from studies of each of these methods are reported. Conclusion—The use of small incisions that produce minimal trauma and preserve most of the blood supply to the periodontal and peri-implant tissues results in improved regenerative outcomes, minimal to absent negative esthetic outcomes, and little or no patient discomfort. Minimally invasive procedures are a reliable method to regenerate periodontal tissues.

Keywords: minimally invasive; videoscope; periodontal surgery; bone regeneration; bone grafts; biologics

1. Literature Review

Periodontal minimally invasive surgery for bone regeneration, termed MIS, was first described by Harrel and Rees in 1995 [1]. The MIS technique was further described in multiple publications from 1995 through 2000 [2–5]. The concepts of minimally invasive surgery for bone regeneration consist of the use of much smaller incisions than those traditionally used for periodontal bone grafting, the maintenance of as much of the blood supply as possible to aid in regeneration and to minimize patient discomfort, and the primary closure of the surgical incisions. At the time MIS was introduced, the visualization of the root surfaces and bony lesions for debridement and placement of demineralized freeze-dried bone allograft (DFDBA) bone grafting material was performed with surgical telescopes (3X to 5X magnification). Because of the challenges of visualization, at this initial stage of MIS surgical technique development, very small buccal and lingual flaps were used. The use of both a buccal and a lingual flap was necessary to allow for adequate visualization of the defect with the telescopes.

The published results of MIS showed excellent improvement in pocket probing depth and attachment level. Multiple case series showed improvements in pocket probing depths of 3 to 5 mm with most post-surgical pocket depths measuring less than 4 mm [2–4]. The long-term post-surgical regenerative results were considered to be equal and, in many cases, superior to the results that were achieved with traditional periodontal bone grafting techniques using a large-flap approach. The patients usually indicated that they had minimal discomfort when MIS was used, but this was not formally measured at that time. However, with the early MIS approach, there was soft tissue recession of one plus mm, which is only slightly less than the amount of recession resulting from traditional surgical approaches.

Harrel and Wilson performed a study using the previously described MIS approach with the addition of enamel matrix derivative (EMD) [6,7]. The flaps, visualization technique, and bone graft with DFDBA were the same as originally described, but, in addition, the manufacturers' recommendation for the use of EMD was followed, and EMD was also added to the DFDBA. Part of the manufacturers' recommendation for the use of EMD is root biomodification with EDTA. This was done for the stated purpose of removing the "smear layer" produced during root planing of the root surface and was designed to allow the EMD to be absorbed into the root surface. The one-year and five-year post-operative data from MIS with EMD were reported on 160 sites. This study showed that excellent results were obtained at one year and that the improvement was maintained for at least five years. The mean improvement in pocket probing depths was 3.50 mm, and the improvement in clinical attachment level (CAL) was 3.48 mm. These results were felt to be an improvement over the results obtained with traditional surgical techniques for bone regeneration. In addition, the post-surgical soft tissue height showed a small mean improvement. With traditional regenerative surgical approaches, a soft tissue loss (recession) of 1–2 mm was reported [8].

While the regenerative results from MIS were considered to be equivalent or improved compared to the regenerative improvements obtained from traditional regenerative surgical approaches, from a clinician and patient satisfaction point of view the results were considered a major improvement over past results. A significant positive feature was the lack of post-surgical recession. Up until these studies, some amount of recession had been reported for all regenerative procedures. The lack of esthetically compromising recession was a new finding.

In 2007, Cortellini and Tonetti published a modification of the original MIS procedure [9]. They termed their procedure the minimally invasive surgery technique (MIST). This procedure used an incision pattern very similar to MIS for access to the bony defect. The major modification of the MIS procedure was that MIST incorporated elements of the papilla preservation technique. These modifications involved the handling of the buccal flap and the suturing technique used to close the surgical site. Where the MIS procedures used a simple vertical mattress suture at the base of the papilla and the incisions were closed with finger pressure, the papilla preservation suturing used in MIST utilized overlapping sutures to approximate the edges of the incision. No bone graft was used in MIST, but EMD was placed in the lesion. Visualization for MIST was obtained using the surgical microscope. The reported results from MIST were very similar to those reported from MIS with EMD. Slightly more recession was noted following MIST (0.4 mm) than with MIS combined with EMD, but recession in both procedures was very minor to non-existent. Further reports by Cortellini and others also showed excellent results [10–14]. A latter change in the MIST procedure, termed modified MIST (M-MIST), was introduced that utilized only a buccal flap [12].

MIS and MIST used very similar incisions and tissue handling to achieve improvements in pocket probing depths and clinical attachment with minimal soft tissue changes. Both procedures yielded results that were equal to or improved over the regenerative results gained with traditional regenerative procedures such as bone grafts or guided tissue regeneration. Despite these excellent and consistent results from two separate research centers, minimally invasive small incision surgery did not become a routine approach for regeneration of bone in periodontal defects. While there are many factors that may have influenced the acceptance of minimally invasive techniques, the difficulty of visualizing the defect through the small openings was probably the leading factor. It can be extremely difficult to visualize the base of a defect or the accretions on a root surface with the technology used in the previously discussed studies, i.e., surgical loops or surgical microscope.

2. Visualization Techniques

The original MIS procedure was performed with relatively high-magnification surgical telescopes with headlights. While this technology is a major improvement over direct visualization, the magnification available was inadequate for very small incisions, and it was frequently necessary to use longer incisions in order to visualize the defect. The use of a surgical microscope, as in MIST, improved the magnification available, but many surgeons find the bulkiness of the microscope to be a negative factor. If any patient movement occurs during a procedure, either the patient or the surgical microscope has to be meticulously repositioned. Another visualization method that was attempted for MIS was the use of a glass fiber flexible endoscope (Periovue) designed for non-surgical use. This device uses a water-filled environment to keep the lens of the endoscope clear. It was found that it was difficult to impossible to keep a surgical site filled with water, which made the use of this endoscope very difficult and time-consuming.

The goal for minimally invasive surgery is to regenerate lost periodontal supporting tissue utilizing the smallest possible incisions and flap openings. In addition, the maintenance or improvement of patient esthetics is a major goal. It became obvious that the visualization technology that had been used in MIS and MIST was inadequate to make the incisions smaller. Also, in order to attain the most esthetic end results, a visualization technology that could be easily used with a lingual approach, as opposed to a buccal approach or a buccal and lingual approach, was necessary. While both telescopes and surgical microscope can be used with a mirror to obtain visualization from the lingual, this extra step can be difficult in many areas of the mouth. The lack of visualization technology that was easy to use in the lingual approach was probably influential in the design of M-MIST where a buccal approach was used for access. An ideal visualization technology needs to be small enough to fit into a very small surgical access, easily maneuverable so the entire bony lesion and adjacent root surface can be easily observed, and capable of delivering good visualization using a single lingual flap.

With these goals in mind, research was undertaken to create a new technology specifically designed for minimally invasive periodontal regenerative procedures. This research was made possible by a grant from the US National Institutes of Health (Bethesda, MD, USA). The result was a surgical videoscope designed for oral use. A videoscope is an instrument that has a very small digital camera that can be inserted directly into the surgical site. The image is transmitted from the camera to a monitor as an electronic signal. This differs from an endoscope in which a lens arrangement is inserted into the surgical site and the image is transmitted to an external camera through a fiber optic bundle. A videoscope is capable of a much clearer and true color picture of the surgical site than a fiber optic endoscope. The transmission of the image through the fiber optic bundle results in significant image degradation so that what is seen on the monitor is unclear and often has a false color. By transmitting an electronic signal, the camera in the videoscope has minimal optical distortion and the colors are more true to life. The surgical videoscope was first described in 2013 [15]. The currently used videoscope is pictured in Figure 1.

Another concern with any optical device placed in a surgical site is the obscuring of the optical lens by blood or surgical debris. When this occurs, the device must be removed from the surgical site, and the lens cleaned. Because the lens becomes obscured very quickly in the small surgical access used for MIS or MIST, it is impossible to use an optical device like a videoscope or endoscope without a method that keeps the lens clean. The dental endoscope used for non-surgical periodontal procedures addresses this problem with a constant flow of water. This is not feasible for a surgical procedure because the water is not adequately contained. In addition, the water adds a distortion to the image seen on the monitor. The videoscope used for minimally invasive surgery solves this problem by passing a stream of low-pressure air over the camera lens. This forms a vortex in front of the camera lens and effectively forces away debris form the lens and keeps the lens free from blood and other debris. The air pressure used is quite low and does not represent a danger of soft tissue emphysema [16].

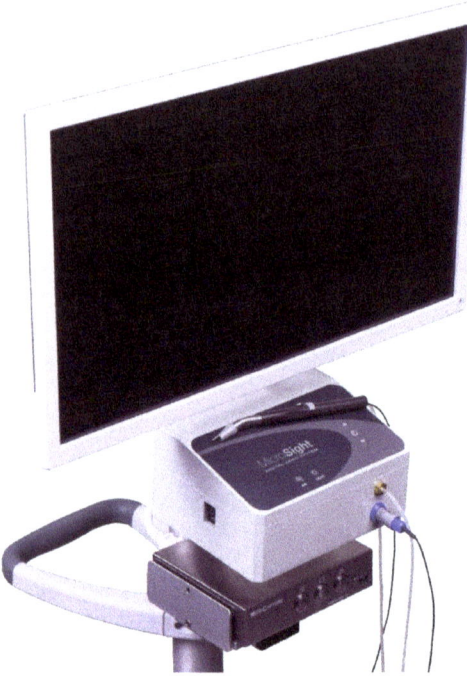

Figure 1. The videoscope designed for oral surgical procedures (MicroSight, Q-Optics, USA).

3. Videoscope-Assisted Minimally Invasive Surgery (VMIS)

Following the development of the videoscope designed for use in minimally invasive periodontal regenerative surgery, a surgical procedure specifically designed to take advantage of the videoscope was developed. The MIS procedure was used as a starting point for the surgical technique that became known as Videoscope-Assisted Minimally Invasive Surgery (VMIS) [17–20]. The procedure is discussed in detail in the paragraphs below.

Indication—The most common situation in which to perform VMIS is for regeneration of bone loss in interproximal areas. Frequently, patients will initially present with generalized moderate to severe periodontitis. Following oral hygiene instruction and non-surgical root planing, most pocket probing depths may return to an acceptable level of 4 mm or less. However, there will frequently be isolated areas of bone loss where the pocket probing depth is unacceptably deep. The interproximal areas are the most frequent location of these deeper areas. With traditional surgery for regeneration, buccal and lingual incisions covering one or two teeth on either side of these isolated defects would be used. These longer incisions are made on periodontally healthy teeth and increase the probability of post-surgical recession and discomfort. With VMIS, incisions are made only in the area of the defect. It is unnecessary to extend the incisions to healthy areas for the sake of visualization. While the videoscope is used for many other surgical procedures beyond these isolated interproximal lesions, VMIS for this type of lesion will be described here.

Incisions—The incisions for VMIS are limited to the area of bone loss. In most cases, the mesial-distal length of the incision is no more than 6–8 mm. With the availability of the videoscope, it is not necessary to use a longer incision to obtain visualization. The incisions are shown in Figure 2.

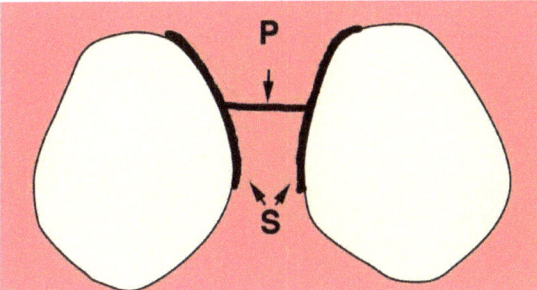

Figure 2. The incisions used for Videoscope-Assisted Minimally Invasive Surgery (VMIS). The incisions are made on the lingual aspect in the area of bone loss. Sulcular incisions (S) are made on the lingual aspect of the teeth adjacent to the area of interproximal bone loss. A split-thickness connecting incision is made at the base of the papilla (P).

A sulcular incision (S in Figure 2) is made on the lingual aspect of the teeth on either side of the area of bone loss. When these incisions are made, the blade is placed against the root surface and inserted to the base of the defect. No tissue is removed with this incision. Unlike more traditional surgical approaches where the sulcus lining is removed or a "collar of tissue" is removed, the goal with VMIS incisions is to sever the granulation tissue only and to leave the rest of the tissue intact. Following the placement of the sulcular incisions, a connecting incision is made at the base of the papilla (P in Figure 2). This incision is made only to the crest of the bone. The goal is to retain as much of the periosteum on the bone as possible. Depending on the anatomy of the area, this may be the full extent of incisions that is necessary. If there is inadequate room to place the soft tissue retractor of the videoscope or if the bony defect cannot be adequately visualized, the papillary incision (P) can be extended apically as a split-thickness incision (Figure 3). Under no circumstance should a periosteal elevator be used to gain space. A periosteal elevator will pull the periosteum from the bone, which will greatly diminish the blood supply to the periodontal tissue. The use of a periosteal elevator is associated with a greater recession than that observed when a split-thickness approach is used.

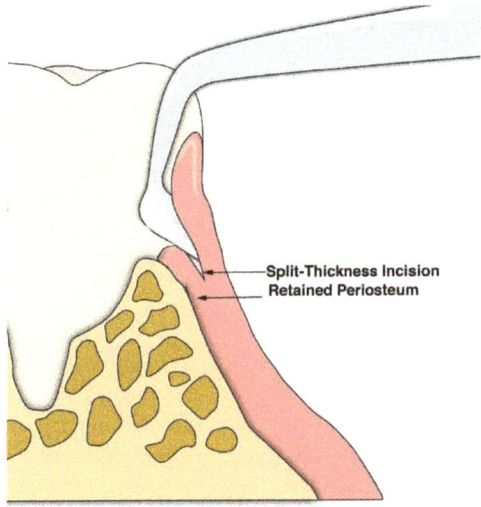

Figure 3. The split-thickness incisions at the base of the papilla (P in Figure 2) are designed to leave the periosteium intact. A periosteal elevator should not be used.

Debridement—Once incisions and the small split-thickness lingual flap have been made, the retractor on the handpiece of the videoscope is inserted, and light pressure is placed on the flap so that the defect can be visualized. Generally, there will be a significant amount of granulation tissue in the defect which must be removed. This is usually performed with a Younger-Goode curette that has been reduced in size by about one-third from its original size. This curette is used in an action similar to using an instrument to "spoon" out caries from a tooth. This action is more suitable for the small flaps of VMIS than the traditional "scaling" action used with surgical curettes. Once the granulation tissue has been removed, the root surfaces can be debrided of accretions and roughness. This is performed with a combination of ultrasonic instrumentation and hand instruments. The videoscope is used throughout the debridement process. When an ultrasonic scaler is used, there will be some transient blurring of the videoscope image due to water on the lens, but the air over the lens clears the image in a matter of seconds when the ultrasonic scaler is turned off. After mechanical debridement of the roots, they are dried with gauze and thoroughly inspected with the videoscope. The 20 to 40× magnification of the videoscope often reveals "micro-islands" of calculus and anatomical roughness on the root surface. [20] These can be removed with the use of EDTA (Prefgel, Straumann, USA), recommended by the manufacturer for the biomodification of the root surface before using EMD. A fully debrided defect ready for bone grafting is shown in Figure 4.

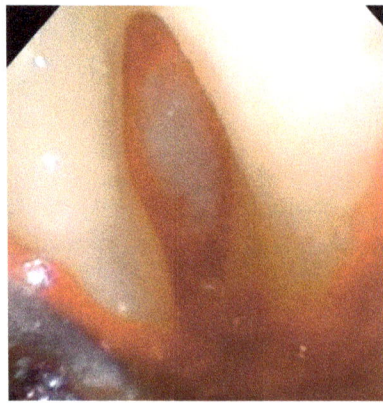

Figure 4. A furcation defect that has been fully debrided and EDTA used to remove any micro-islands of calculus. This site is ready for bone grafting and enamel matrix derivative (EMD) treatment.

Bone Graft—Following the use of EDTA to remove any remaining micro-islands of calculus, the defect is rinsed, and EMD is placed on the root surface. The remaining EMD is mixed with DFDBA or other bone grafting material and gently placed into the bony defect. The defect should not be overfilled, as that will potentially interfere with the ability to obtain primary closure of the soft tissue. Membranes are never used in VMIS. The incisions would have to be greatly expanded to accommodate a membrane, and the use of a membrane is unnecessary to achieve the results reported in the literature for VMIS.

Suturing—A single vertical mattress suture placed at the base of the papilla is recommended for each site of VMIS. It is not necessary to use the papilla preservation suturing technique when the VMIS incision pattern is used. The suture should be placed in the thick area of tissue at the base of the papilla. No sutures are placed directly at the connecting incision between the two teeth. It has been determined that placing sutures in this thin tissue leads to greater post-operative recession. Once the single suture is placed at the base of the papilla, the incisions are primarily approximated by using finger pressure on a saline-soaked gauze. A closed surgical site is shown in Figure 5.

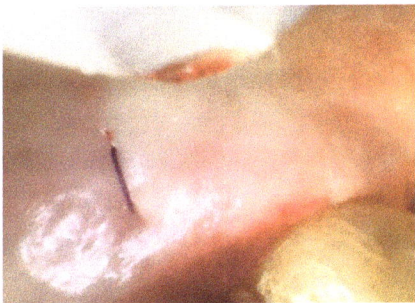

Figure 5. A Videoscope-Assisted Minimally Invasive Surgery (VMIS) palatal flap closed with a single vertical mattress suture at the base of the papilla. The edges of the incision in the papilla have been approximated with finger pressure only.

The surgical technique described above was utilized in a masked outcome-based case series of 30 patients and 110 sites. The surgical sites in this study were areas of pocket probing depth of 5mm or greater at six weeks post root planing that also had radiographic evidence of bone loss and no greater than a class-I furcation defect. The results from this case series were reported at six months, one year, and 3 to 5 years post-surgery [17–20]. Statistically significant improvements in pocket probing depth (3.8 mm), clinical attachment levels (4.16 mm), and soft tissue height (0.38 mm) were noted at all measurement intervals and were stable for the 3- to 5-year time period. All surgical sites were noted to be less than 4 mm at 5 years post-surgery, with a mean pocket probing depth of less than 3 mm.

Discomfort and patient satisfaction—Patient pain levels were evaluated on the day of surgery and at each follow-up appointment. Two patients indicated very slight discomfort on the day of surgery, one patient had slight discomfort one week post-surgery. With these exceptions, no patient reported any discomfort at any time following VMIS. All patients indicated satisfaction with the surgical procedure, satisfaction with the esthetic outcomes, and would have the procedure done again at another site if indicated. It should be noted that, in this long-term study, there was no mean recession in the surgical sites and there was a mean improvement in soft tissue height of nearly 0.5 mm, which contributed to patient satisfaction with esthetics. Both lack of recession and soft tissue improvement have not been reported with any other periodontal bone regenerative procedure.

4. VMIS for Peri-Implant Bone Loss

The VMIS procedure has been modified for regeneration in areas of bone loss on implants. The results from this new approach have been encouraging. A study is underway on this approach but has not been completed.

The cause of bone loss around implants is unknown, and many different causes for bone loss around implants may exist. Clearly, because the implant interface with the bone is completely different from a natural tooth, it is unlikely that peri-implant bone loss is the same process that occurs in periodontal bone loss around natural teeth. Various factors have been suggested, including bacterial plaque, occlusion, and improper surgical placement of the implants. Wilson et al. showed that there were multiple particles of both titanium and cement embedded in the soft tissue surrounding many failed implants, and these particles were always surrounded by inflammatory cells [21]. The localized inflammatory response universally noted around these particles resembles a foreign body reaction seen with other materials. This phenomenon has led to the hypothesis that, in addition to excess cement, bone loss around implants may be associated with a foreign body reaction to titanium particles from the implant caused by corrosion or other stresses on the implant surface. The use of the VMIS procedure for treating implant bone loss is specifically aimed at removing any particles of cement or titanium that may be embedded in the implant soft tissue and potentially contributing to a pathologic foreign body reaction.

The incisions used are very similar to those previously described for VMIS around natural teeth. A sulcular incision is made around the implant in the area of bone loss. No soft tissue is removed at this point. The incision is extended apically to the level of remaining bone. A split-thickness incision is then made across the base of the adjoining papilla extending to the line angle of the adjacent teeth. As with natural teeth, the split-thickness incision is extended apically for an adequate distance to allow for the insertion of the retractor tip on the videoscope and to allow adequate visualization of the bone loss. (Figure 6).

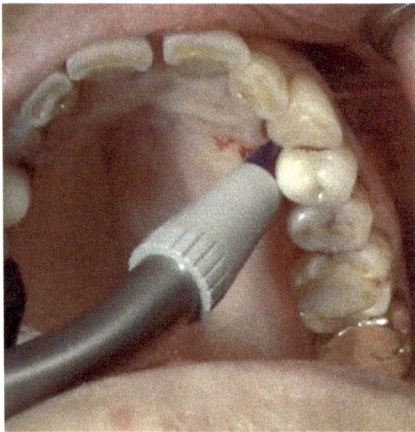

Figure 6. The tip of the retractor on the videoscope is rotated to an optimal angle and used to gently push back the lingual flap to allow visualization of the bone loss.

Once the implant has been adequately visualized, under videoscope guidance and using a new small blade, a thin section of tissue approximately 1–2 mm in thickness is removed from the tissue that was in contact with the implant in the area of bone loss. (Figure 7) When this tissue is evaluated histologically, as was done in the study by Wilson et al., multiple areas of cement and/or titanium particles surrounded by inflammatory cells are often noted. The purpose of removing this tissue is to eliminate foreign material that may cause further damage to the implant-supporting bone in the future as well as may interfere with the regeneration of bone around the implant.

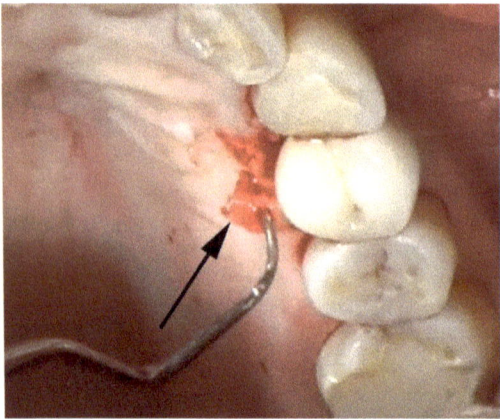

Figure 7. A thin (1–2 mm) section of tissue (arrow) containing foreign particles of titanium or cement is removed from the area of bone loss.

Following the removal of the thin section of tissue, any granulation tissue is removed in a similar manner as performed on natural teeth. However, care should be taken to not touch the implant surface with the instrument used to remove the granulation tissue. The implant surface is covered by titanium oxide, and this has been shown to be an integral part of the osseointegration process [22]. Titanium oxide is very fragile and will be damaged or corroded if the implant surface is touched by an instrument or disinfected with harsh chemicals such as citric acid or a tetracycline solution. Because of this, great care is taken to not touch the implant with a curette while removing the granulation tissue and to only gently wipe the implant surface with sterile gauze soaked in saline. The debrided peri-implant bone loss is shown in Figure 8.

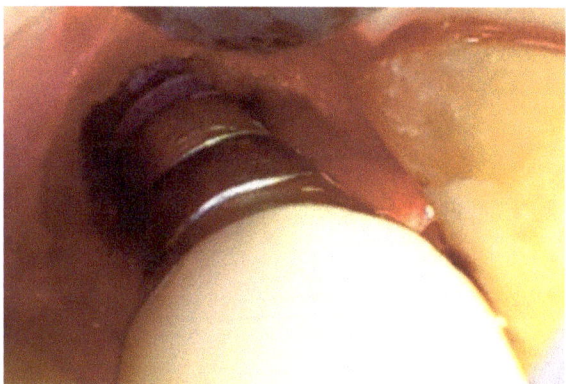

Figure 8. The fully debrided bony lesion can be visualized after removal of the granulation tissue.

After the lesion is debrided of granulation tissue and the implant is cleaned with saline, DFDBA mixed with EMD is place in the bony defect. (Figure 9).

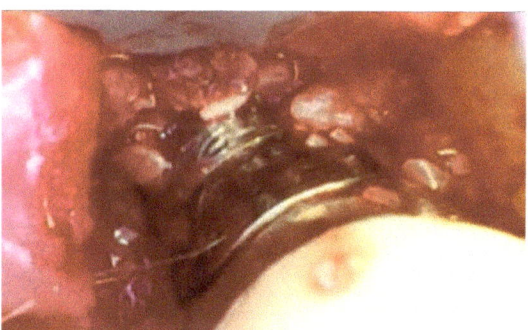

Figure 9. The bony lesion pictured in Figure 8 has been filled with particulate bone-grafting material mixed with EMD.

EDTA is not burnished on the surface of the implant. Radiographs taken one year post-surgery appear to show bone formation in the area of initial bone loss. Further, it appears that the new bone has formed in contact with the implant surface. The frequently seen "black line" between the implant and newly formed bone is not present. The lack of a black line may be an indication of re-osseointegration. However, this can only be proven with a block biopsy of the implant and bone. This type of biopsy is not ethically acceptable with a clinically functional implant, so the existence of re-osseointegration remains a conjecture.

5. Summary

The existing literature on minimally invasive periodontal surgery, the literature on the videoscope, the literature on VMIS, and the techniques designed around the advantages of the videoscope have been reviewed. The published clinical results are favorable and indicate that VMIS can be used to consistently regenerate bone around periodontally damaged teeth with no recession and a possible improvement in soft tissue height. In addition, the application of the VMIS technique to peri-implant bone loss has been reviewed. The videoscope is also being used for other surgical and non-surgical procedures. Some of these are surgical and non-surgical endodontic procedures (Figure 10), sinus elevation surgery (Figure 11), and non-surgical hygiene procedures. Research in these applications is ongoing.

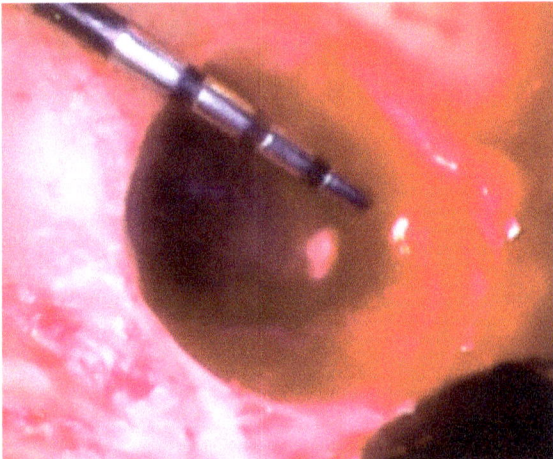

Figure 10. Videoscope visualization of the apex of a maxillary incisor during surgical endodontic treatment.

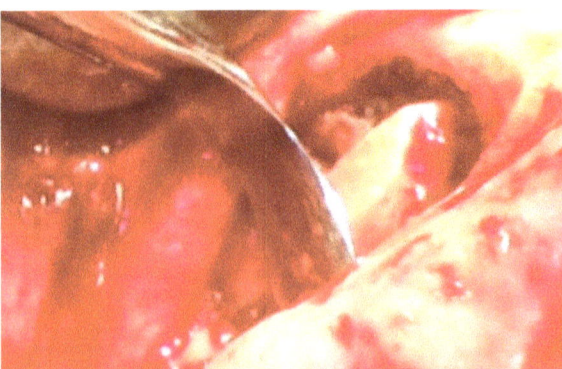

Figure 11. Videoscope visualization of a lateral window access for sinus bone grafting in preparation for placing implants.

Patents—Dr. Harrel holds the patent for the videoscope used in VMIS.

Conflicts of Interest: The author declares no conflict of interest.

References

1. Harrel, S.K.; Rees, T.D. Granulation tissue removal in routine and minimally invasive surgical procedures. *Compend. Contin. Educ. Dent.* **1995**, *16*, 960–967. [PubMed]
2. Harrel, S.K. A minimally invasive surgical approach for bone grafting. *Int. J. Periodont. Rest. Dent.* **1998**, *18*, 161–169.
3. Harrel, S.K. A minimally invasive surgical approach for periodontal regeneration: Surgical technique and observations. *J. Periodontol.* **1999**, *70*, 1547–1557. [CrossRef] [PubMed]
4. Harrel, S.K.; Nunn, M.; Belling, C.M. Long-term results of a minimally invasive surgical approach for bone grafting. *J. Periodontol.* **1999**, *70*, 1558–1563. [CrossRef] [PubMed]
5. Harrel, S.K.; Wright, J.M. Treatment of periodontal destruction associated with a cemental tear using minimally invasive surgery. *J. Periodontol.* **2000**, *71*, 1761–1766. [CrossRef] [PubMed]
6. Harrel, S.K.; Wilson, T.G.; Nunn, M.E. Prospective assessment of the use of enamel matrix proteins with minimally invasive surgery. *J. Periodontol.* **2005**, *76*, 380–384. [CrossRef] [PubMed]
7. Harrel, S.K.; Wilson, T.G.; Nunn, M.E. Prospective assessment of the use of enamel matrix derivative with minimally invasive surgery: Six year results. *J. Periodontol.* **2010**, *81*, 435–444. [CrossRef] [PubMed]
8. Garrett, S. Periodontal regeneration around natural teeth. *Ann. Periodontal* **1996**, *1*, 621–666. [CrossRef] [PubMed]
9. Cortellini, P.; Tonetti, M.S. A minimally invasive surgical technique with an enamel matrix derivative in the regenerative treatment of intra-bony defects: A novel approach to limit morbidity. *J. Clin. Periodontol.* **2007**, *34*, 87–93. [CrossRef] [PubMed]
10. Cortellini, P.; Tonetti, M.S. Minimally invasive surgical technique and enamel matrix derivative in intra-bony defects. I: Clinical outcomes and morbidity. *J. Clin. Periodontol.* **2007**, *34*, 1082–1088. [CrossRef] [PubMed]
11. Cortellini, P.; Nieri, M.; Prato, G.P.; Tonetti, M.S. Single minimally invasive surgical technique with an enamel matrix derivative to treat multiple adjacent intra-bony defects: Clinical outcomes and patient morbidity. *J. Clin. Periodontol.* **2008**, *35*, 605–613. [CrossRef] [PubMed]
12. Cortellini, P.; Tonetti, M.S. Improved wound stability with a modified minimally invasive surgical technique in the regenerative treatment of isolated interdental intrabony defects. *J. Clin. Periodontol.* **2009**, *36*, 157–163. [CrossRef] [PubMed]
13. Cortellini, P.; Pino-Prato, G.; Nieri, M.; Tonetti, M.S. Minimally invasive surgical technique and enamel matrix derivative in intrabony pocket: 2 Factors associated with healing outcomes. *Int. J. Periodont. Restor. Dent.* **2009**, *29*, 257–265.
14. Cortellini, P.; Tonetti, M.S. Clinical and radiographic outcomes of the modified minimally invasive surgical technique with and without regenerative materials: A randomized-controlled trial in intra-bony defects. *J. Clin. Periodontol.* **2011**, *38*, 365–373. [CrossRef] [PubMed]
15. Harrel, S.K.; Wilson, T.G., Jr.; Rivera-Hidalgo, F. A videoscope for use in minimally invasive periodontal surgery. *J. Clin. Periodontol.* **2013**, *40*, 868–874. [CrossRef] [PubMed]
16. Harrel, S.K.; Rivera-Hidalgo, F.; Abraham, C. Tissue Resistance to Soft Tissue Emphysema during Minimally Invasive Surgery. *J. Contemp. Dent. Pract.* **2012**, *13*, 886–891. [CrossRef] [PubMed]
17. Harrel, S.K.; Abraham, C.M.; Rivera-Hidalgo, F.; Shulman, J.; Nunn, M. Videoscope-assisted minimally invasive periodontal surgery (V-MIS). *J. Clin. Periodontol.* **2014**, *41*, 900–907. [CrossRef] [PubMed]
18. Harrel, S.K.; Rivera-Hidalgo, F.; Shulman, J.; Nunn, M. Videoscope Assisted Minimally Invasive Periodontal Surgery: One Year Outcome and Patient Morbidity. *Int. J. Periodont. Rest. Dent.* **2016**, *36*, 363–371. [CrossRef] [PubMed]
19. Harrel, S.K.; Nunn, M.E.; Abraham, C.M.; Rivera-Hidalgo, F.; Shulman, J.D.; Tunnell, J.C. Videoscope Assisted Minimally Invasive Surgery (VMIS): 36-Month Results. *J. Periodontol.* **2017**, *88*, 528–535. [CrossRef] [PubMed]
20. Harrel, S.K.; Valderrama, P.; Barnes, J.B.; Blackwell, E.L. Frequency of root surface microgrooves associated with periodontal destruction. *Int. J. Periodont. Restor. Dent.* **2016**, *36*, 841–846. [CrossRef] [PubMed]

21. Wilson, T.G., Jr.; Valderrama, P.; Burbano, M.; Blansett, J.; Levine, R.; Kessler, H.; Rodrigues, D.C. Foreign bodies associated with peri-implantitis human biopsies. *J. Periodontol.* **2015**, *86*, 9–15. [CrossRef] [PubMed]
22. Sul, Y.-T. On the Bone Response to Oxidized Titanium Implants: The Role of Microporous Structure and Chemical Composition of the Surface Oxide in Enhanced Osseointegration. Ph.D. Thesis, University of Gothenburg, Göteborg, Sweden, 2002.

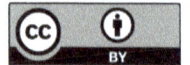

© 2018 by the author. Licensee MDPI, Basel, Switzerland. This article is an open access article distributed under the terms and conditions of the Creative Commons Attribution (CC BY) license (http://creativecommons.org/licenses/by/4.0/).

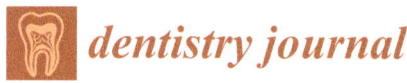

Case Report

Combination Therapy for Reconstructive Periodontal Treatment in the Lower Anterior Area: Clinical Evaluation of a Case Series

Carlos E. Nemcovsky * and Ilan Beitlitum

Department of Periodontology and Dental Implantology Dental School, Tel-Aviv University, Tel Aviv 6139001, Israel; beilan@post.tau.ac.il
* Correspondence: carlos@post.tau.ac.il; Tel.: +972-5-4462-6345

Received: 27 August 2018; Accepted: 20 September 2018; Published: 1 October 2018

Abstract: Clinically, periodontal regeneration may be achieved by the application of barrier membranes, grafts, wound-healing modifiers, and their combinations. Combination therapy refers to the simultaneous application of various periodontal reconstructive treatment alternatives to obtain additive effects. This approach may lead to assemblage of different regenerative principles, such as conductivity and inductivity, space provision and wound stability, matrix development and cell differentiation. The application of autogenous connective tissue grafts during periodontal regenerative treatment with enamel matrix proteins derivative (EMD) has been previously reported. The present case series present a modified approach for treatment of severe periodontally involved lower incisors presenting with thin gingival biotype, gingival recession, minimal attached and keratinized gingiva width and muscle and/or frenum pull. In all cases a combination therapy consisting of a single buccal access flap, root conditioning, EMD application on the denuded root surfaces and a free connective tissue graft was performed. Clinical and radiographic outcomes were consistently satisfactory, leading to probing depth reduction, clinical attachment gain, minimal gingival recession, increased attached and keratinizing gingival width, elimination of frenum and/or muscle pull together with radiographic bone fill of the defects. It may be concluded that the present combination therapy for reconstructive periodontal treatment in the lower anterior area is a valuable alternative for indicated cases.

Keywords: periodontal regeneration; connective tissue graft; enamel matrix proteins derivative; root coverage; combination therapy; soft tissue management; periodontal surgery

1. Introduction

Reconstructive periodontal procedures improve tooth survival while reducing periodontitis progression and re-intervention needs providing long-term outcome stability [1]. Provided adequate periodontal treatment and maintenance, even with reduced periodontal attachment level, natural dentition yields better long-term survival and marginal bone level changes compared with dental implants [2].

Periodontal reconstruction is a complex biological process that involves de novo formation of the lost tooth supporting structures, including alveolar bone, periodontal ligament, and cementum over a previously diseased root surface.

Reconstructive periodontal procedures have shown advantages over conventional surgical procedures in terms of better results in long-term stability, improved tooth survival, less periodontitis progression and fewer needs for re-intervention over long periods [1].

In addition, certain delivery agents have been proven to improve the efficacy of non-surgical periodontal therapy [3–5]. Clinically, periodontal regeneration may be achieved by application of barrier membranes, grafts, wound-healing modifiers, and their combinations.

Guided tissue regeneration (GTR) is based on the application of a separating barrier membrane mechanically isolating the defect. Although this mechanical/biological concept has been widely proven both in pre-clinical and clinical studies, several shortcomings such as treatment of multiple proximal defects, complications due to membrane exposure and recessions of the neighboring teeth [6,7] and incomplete adaptation of the membrane around irregularly shaped roots, has limited their application in regenerative periodontal surgical procedures.

Enamel matrix protein derivatives (EMD) are the most largely evaluated in both pre-clinical [8] and clinical models, mainly composed of amelogenins, with smaller amounts of other non-amelogenin components, such as tuftelin, ameloblastin and enamel proteases [9]. EMD is a biologically active compound that, once applied on a denuded root surface, starts a cascade of biological events, such as enhanced attraction and migration of mesenchymal cells, their attachment to the root surface [10] and, differentiation into cementoblasts, PDL fibroblasts and osteoblasts. Enamel proteins enhance gene expression responsible for protein and mineralized tissue syntheses in PDL cells [11]. This process may finally lead to reconstitution of the periodontal apparatus.

Application of EMD during reconstructive periodontal surgical therapy enhanced the outcome in respect to clinical attachment level (CAL) gain, probing pocket depth reduction, and new bone formation, compared with open-flap debridement and/or modified Widman flap [6,7,12–15].

Due to a lesser gingival recession, EMD treatment seems indicated for aesthetic regions. EMD treatment presents less patient morbidity than GTR as membrane exposure occurs in the vast majority of cases treated with GTR, while only few complications occur in EMD treated sites. EMD is a valuable treatment alternative for treating multiple proximal defects without reducing the blood nourishment of the flap leading to extensive membrane exposure. Periodontal regenerative surgery with GTR seems questionable in suprabony defects with horizontal bone loss [16,17], however, EMD application may enhance treatment outcome in these defects [18–21]. Enhanced clinical wound healing rates following EMD treatment may be appreciated. EMD improved oral mucosa incisional wound healing by promoting the formation of blood vessels and collagen fibres in the connective tissue [22]. The increase in soft-tissue density was faster following EMD application compared to the access flap [23].

EMD enhances gingival fibroblasts proliferation [24–29] and positively affects the inflammatory and healing responses by different cellular mechanisms [30–32].

2. Soft Tissue Considerations

Soft tissue management is one of the most important factors for successful outcomes of periodontal reconstructive surgical treatments. Initially, flap designs were based on conventional periodontal procedures. Later, techniques evolved towards soft tissue preservation to achieve and maintain passive primary closure together with optimal wound stability over the regenerative materials, which is critical especially during the initial healing stages [33,34].

The single flap approach provides access to the surgical site by elevation of a single, either buccal or lingual/palatal full-thickness flap [35–40]. The interproximal supracrestal gingival tissues are left intact, allowing for easy flap repositioning with stable primary wound closure. Increased post-surgery gingival recession usually occurs where deep intraosseous are associated with buccal dehiscence defects. The combination of a bioactive agent and a graft material together with a single flap approach may limit postoperative gingival recession [35–40].

3. Combination Therapies

Combination therapy refers to the simultaneous application of various periodontal reconstructive treatment alternatives to obtain an additive effect. This approach may lead to the assemblage of different regenerative principles, such as conductivity and inductivity, space provision and wound stability, matrix development and cell differentiation.

EMD alone, as a single therapy, may be applied mainly in narrow defects with a prevalent three-wall morphology or in well-supported two-wall defects, biomaterials provide soft tissue support, especially in non-self-contained defects. A large access flap may not provide proper wound stability, which may be achieved with barriers or fillers, combinations of barriers and fillers, or combinations of amelogenins and fillers. The combination of a graft biomaterial with biological agents, including EMD, may reduce the post-surgery recession following surgical treatment accessed with the single flap approach [41].

In most types of defects, application of bone grafting material together with EMD led to additional clinical improvements in CAL gain and PD reduction compared with those obtained with EMD alone [42–44].

Periodontal regeneration is the full reconstitution of the lost periodontal support; therefore, application of non-resorbable biomaterials (such as most xenografts) will not lead to true periodontal regeneration.

4. Free Connective Tissue Grafts in Periodontal Regenerative Procedures

Another type of combination therapy is the application of autogenous connective tissue grafts during periodontal reconstructive treatment with EMD [18,19,45]. Histological evaluation of combining a connective tissue graft with EMD in humans has shown varying results, including formation of new cementum, new attachment, and new bone formation after treatment [46,47]. EMD has an enhancing effect on gingival fibroblasts, by increasing up to two-fold, both their proliferation and amount of matrix produced by these cells [24–29] and positively affects the inflammatory and healing responses by different cellular mechanisms [30–32]. Thus, besides the possible periodontal regeneration induction on the denuded root surface, EMD will also enhance the vitality of the free connective tissue graft. During periodontal reconstructive surgery, in cases with minimal amounts of keratinized tissue and in thin periodontal biotypes, a connective tissue can be applied after EMD application onto the denuded root surfaces [20]. This procedure is intended to reduce post-operative gingival recession and increase the gingival dimensions in the area. The beneficial effect of CTG may partly reside in the increase in gingival thickness providing support for the buccal flap. Thick gingival tissues show greater resistance to recession due to surgical trauma and tissue remodelling following different surgical procedures, including regenerative surgery. It may also be speculated that the conversion from a thin to a thick phenotype may have a beneficial effect on the long-term stability of the gingival profile, since thick biotypes were shown to be less prone to developing gingival recessions [48,49].

5. Materials and Methods

The present report is a retrospective evaluation of a surgical procedure performed according to indications. This report includes a series of cases where a modified approach for treatment of severe periodontally involved lower incisors, presenting with thin gingival biotype, gingival recession, minimal attached and keratinized gingiva width and muscle and/or frenum pull, was performed. All cases were treated with a combination therapy consisting of a single buccal access flap, root conditioning, EMD application on the denuded root surfaces and an autogenous free connective tissue graft (Figures 1–8). All patients gave proper informed consent agreeing that the data and clinical evidence be made public through publishing provided their identity was not revealed.

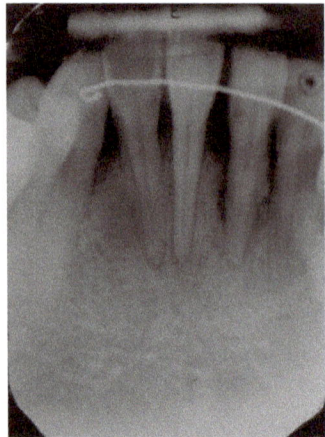

Figure 1. Pre-operative radiograph of lower anterior area showing reduced bone support, with mainly horizontal bone loss.

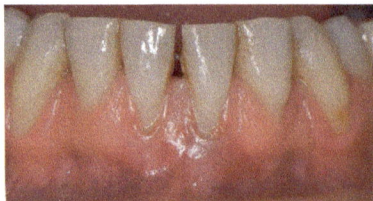

Figure 2. Pre-operative aspect of lower incisors presenting thin gingival biotype, gingival recession, minimal attached and keratinized gingiva width and muscle and frenum pull.

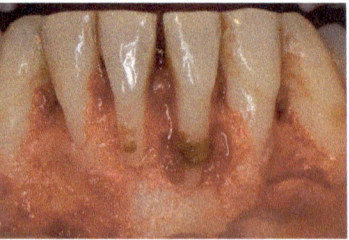

Figure 3. Approach was achieved by raising a single buccal flap, calculus on the denuded root surfaces and large loss of periodontal support are evident.

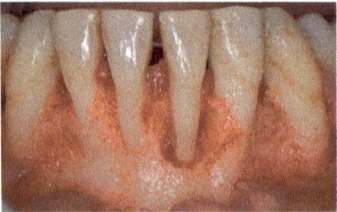

Figure 4. Intra operative aspect, all four lower incisors present extensive root exposure with advanced bone loss, mainly horizontal.

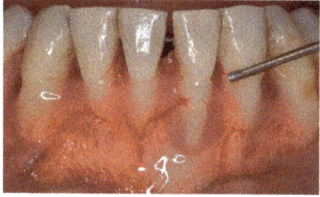

Figure 5. Following root surface conditioning with EDTA gel in a neutral pH for 2 min, enamel maytix proteins derivative gel (EMD) was applied onto denuded root surfaces.

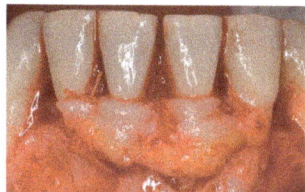

Figure 6. Following EMD application a connective tissue graft was retrieved from the patient's palate and secured covering the denuded root surfaces.

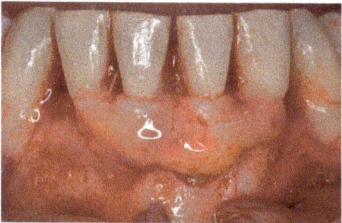

Figure 7. EMD was applied also on top of the soft tissue graft.

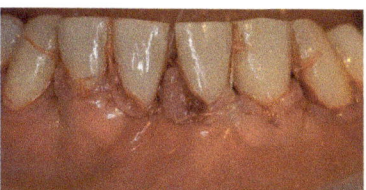

Figure 8. The single buccal flap was coronally displaced and sutured. Tenting sutures were also placed coronally to the contact area to further stabilize the buccal tissues.

6. Results

Clinical and radiographic outcomes were consistently satisfactory leading to probing depth reduction, clinical attachment gain minimal gingival recession, increased attached and keratinizing gingival width, with no frenum and muscle pull together with radiographic bone fill of the defects. Provided there was good supportive periodontal therapy, results were stable for long periods (Figures 9–15).

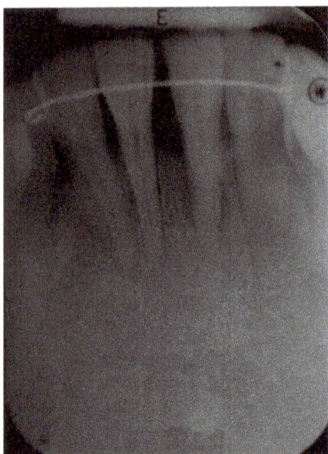

Figure 9. Six-months post-operative radiograph, improved bone support, especially around the central left incisor can already be appreciated.

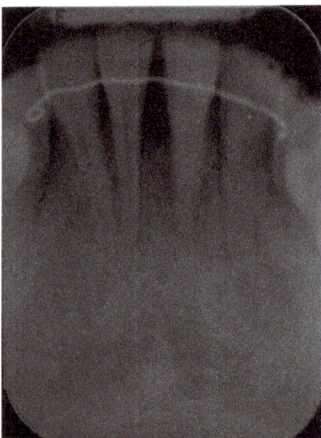

Figure 10. One-year post-operative radiograph, improvement in bone support, especially around the central left incisor is evident, compared to the pre-operative x-ray, the bone defect around the left central incisor has largely been reduced.

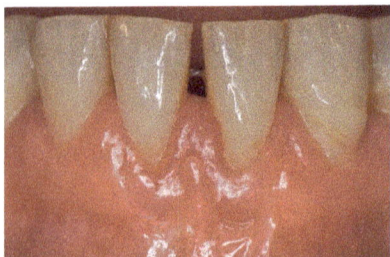

Figure 11. One-year post-operative aspect of lower anterior area. Note gingival aspect, with minimal recession compared to pre-operative aspect, increased attached and keratinized gingival width, with no frenum and muscle pull.

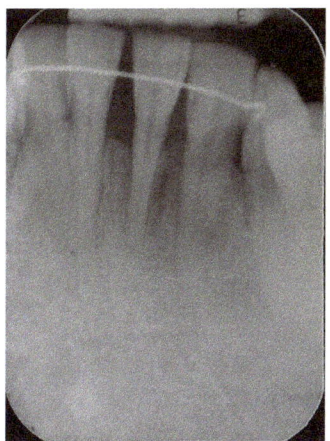

Figure 12. Two-year post-operative radiograph, stable results compared to the one-year situation are evident.

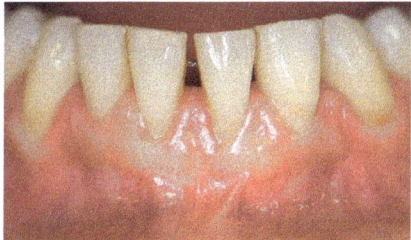

Figure 13. Two-year post-operative aspect of lower anterior area. Note improved gingival aspect, a certain degree of root coverage together with increased attached and keratinized gingival width.

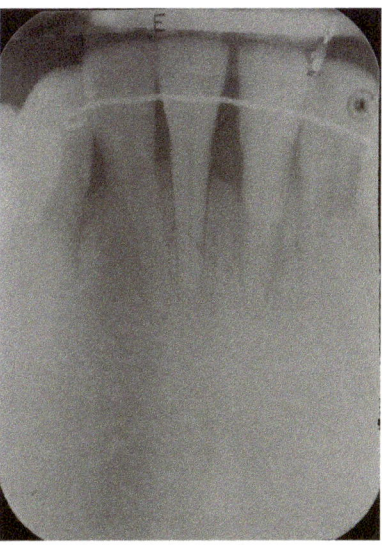

Figure 14. Three years postoperative radiograph, stable results over time can be appreciated.

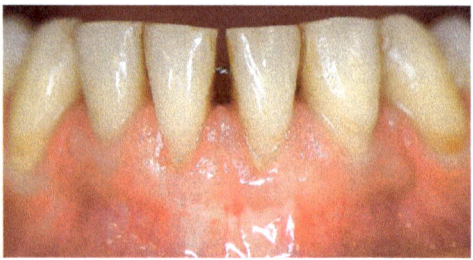

Figure 15. Three-year postoperative aspect of lower anterior area shows stable results over time.

7. Discussion

In the present report, the single flap approach was combined with an autologous soft tissue graft [48,49] in the lower anterior area. Improved clinical outcomes in terms of both defect resolution, reduction of postoperative gingival recession (or even root coverage) and increase in gingival dimensions in addition to a substantial CAL gain especially for deep intraosseous lesions associated with buccal bone dehiscences, as well as challenging intraosseous defects associated with Miller's class IV gingival recession, have been reported [20,48–50]. Varying degrees of gingival recession are usually appreciated following periodontal surgical treatment; the present approach lead to limited or no post-operative recession. Although the present procedure could also be applied in aesthetic areas to reduce gingival recession following treatment, in the present study it was only applied in the lower anterior area with minimal aesthetic relevance.

The adjunctive use of a CTG unavoidably results in a more technically demanding procedure, and increases the intra- and post-operative morbidity due to the need for an additional surgical site for graft harvesting. The addition of connective tissue grafts to periodontal regenerative surgical procedures seems to be particularly beneficial at defects with thin gingival tissues and severe buccal bone dehiscence, usually in the lower anterior area, however, it is of limited relevance in thick biotypes and shallow buccal dehiscences.

8. Conclusions

The combination therapy for reconstructive periodontal treatment in the lower anterior area was able to successfully treat severe periodontally involved lower incisors presenting with thin gingival biotype, gingival recession, minimal attached and keratinized gingiva width and muscle and/or frenum pull. The outcomes showed probing depth reduction, clinical attachment gain minimal gingival recession, increased attached and keratinizing gingival width, with no frenum and muscle pull together with radiographic bone fill of the defects.

Author Contributions: Conceptualization, C.E.N. and I.B.; Methodology, C.E.N.; Validation, C.E.N. and I.B.; Writing-Original Draft Preparation, C.E.N.; Writing-Review & Editing, C.E.N. and I.B.

Funding: The present evaluation neither required nor received any type of funding.

Conflicts of Interest: Authors declare no conflicts of interest.

References

1. Cortellini, P.; Buti, J.; Pini Prato, G.; Tonetti, M.S. Periodontal regeneration compared with access flap surgery in human intra-bony defects 20-year follow-up of a randomized clinical trial: Tooth retention, periodontitis recurrence and costs. *J. Clin. Periodontol.* **2017**, *44*, 58–66. [CrossRef] [PubMed]
2. Rasperini, G.; Siciliano, V.I.; Cafiero, C.; Salvi, G.E.; Blasi, A.; Aglietta, M. Crestal bone changes at teeth and implants in periodontally healthy and periodontally compromised patients. A 10-year comparative case-series study. *J. Periodontol.* **2014**, *85*, e152–e159. [CrossRef] [PubMed]

3. Isola, G.; Matarese, G.; Williams, R.C.; Siciliano, V.I.; Alibrandi, A.; Cordasco, G.; Ramaglia, L. The effects of a desiccant agent in the treatment of chronic periodontitis: A randomized, controlled clinical trial. *Clin. Oral Investig.* **2018**, *22*, 791–800. [CrossRef] [PubMed]
4. Tabenski, L.; Moder, D.; Cieplik, F.; Schenke, F.; Hiller, K.A.; Buchalla, W.; Schmalz, G.; Christgau, M. Antimicrobial photodynamic therapy vs. local minocycline in addition to non-surgical therapy of deep periodontal pockets: A controlled randomized clinical trial. *Clin. Oral Investig.* **2017**, *21*, 2253–2264. [CrossRef] [PubMed]
5. Matarese, G.; Ramaglia, L.; Cicciù, M.; Cordasco, G.; Isola, G. The Effects of Diode Laser Therapy as an Adjunct to Scaling and Root Planing in the Treatment of Aggressive Periodontitis: A 1-Year Randomized Controlled Clinical Trial. *Photomed. Laser Surg.* **2017**, *35*, 702–709. [CrossRef] [PubMed]
6. Esposito, M.; Coulthard, P.; Thomsen, P.; Worthington, H.V. Enamel matrix derivative for periodontal tissue regeneration in treatment of intrabony defects: A cochrane systematic review. *J. Dent. Educ.* **2004**, *68*, 834–844. [PubMed]
7. Sanz, M.; Tonetti, M.S.; Zabalegui, I.; Sicilia, A.; Blanco, J.; Rebelo, H.; Rasperini, G.; Merli, M.; Cortellini, P.; Suvan, J.E. Treatment of intrabony defects with enamel matrix proteins or barrier membranes: Results from a multicenter practice-based clinical trial. *J. Periodontol.* **2004**, *75*, 726–733. [CrossRef] [PubMed]
8. Weinreb, M.; Nemcovsky, C.E. In vitro models for evaluation of periodontal wound healing/regeneration. *Periodontol. 2000* **2015**, *68*, 41–54. [CrossRef] [PubMed]
9. Zeichner-David, M. Is there more to enamel matrix proteins than biomineralization? *Matrix Boil. J. Int. Soc. Matrix Boil.* **2001**, *20*, 307–316. [CrossRef]
10. Rincon, J.C.; Xiao, Y.; Young, W.G.; Bartold, P.M. Enhanced proliferation, attachment and osteopontin expression by porcine periodontal cells exposed to emdogain. *Arch. Oral Boil.* **2005**, *50*, 1047–1054. [CrossRef]
11. Barkana, I.; Alexopoulou, E.; Ziv, S.; Jacob-Hirsch, J.; Amariglio, N.; Pitaru, S.; Vardimon, A.D.; Nemcovsky, C.E. Gene profile in periodontal ligament cells and clones with enamel matrix proteins derivative. *J. Clin. Periodontol.* **2007**, *34*, 599–609. [CrossRef] [PubMed]
12. Heijl, L.; Heden, G.; Svardstrom, G.; Ostgren, A. Enamel matrix derivative (emdogain) in the treatment of intrabony periodontal defects. *J. Clin. Periodontol.* **1997**, *24*, 705–714. [CrossRef] [PubMed]
13. Sculean, A.; Chiantella, G.C.; Windisch, P.; Donos, N. Clinical and histologic evaluation of human intrabony defects treated with an enamel matrix protein derivative (emdogain). *Int. J. Periodontics Restor. Dent.* **2000**, *20*, 374–381.
14. Venezia, E.; Goldstein, M.; Boyan, B.D.; Schwartz, Z. The use of enamel matrix derivative in the treatment of periodontal defects: A literature review and meta-analysis. *Crit. Rev. Oral Boil. Med. Off. Publ. Am. Assoc. Oral Boil.* **2004**, *15*, 382–402. [CrossRef]
15. Francetti, L.; Trombelli, L.; Lombardo, G.; Guida, L.; Cafiero, C.; Roccuzzo, M.; Carusi, G.; Del Fabbro, M. Evaluation of efficacy of enamel matrix derivative in the treatment of intrabony defects: A 24-month multicenter study. *Int. J. Periodontics Restor. Dent.* **2005**, *25*, 461–473.
16. Flores-de-Jacoby, L.; Zimmermann, A.; Tsalikis, L. Experiences with guided tissue regeneration in the treatment of advanced periodontal disease. A clinical re-entry study. Part I. Vertical, horizontal and horizontal periodontal defects. *J. Clin. Periodontol.* **1994**, *21*, 113–117. [CrossRef] [PubMed]
17. Warrer, K.; Karring, T. Guided tissue regeneration combined with osseous grafting in suprabony periodontal lesions. An experimental study in the dog. *J. Clin. Periodontol.* **1992**, *19*, 373–380. [CrossRef] [PubMed]
18. Nemcovsky, C.E. Chapter 12: Clinical applications and techniques in regenerative periodontal therapy. In *Periodontal Regenerative Therapy*; Sculean, A., Ed.; Quintessence International Publishing Co.: Batavia, IL, USA, 2010; pp. 159–193.
19. Nemcovsky, C.E.; Sculean, A. Chapter: Evidence-Based Decision Making in Periodontal Tooth Prognosis and Maintenance of the Natural Dentition. In *Evidence-Based Decision Making in Dentistry. Multidisciplinary Management of the Natural Dentition*; Rosen, E., Nemcovsky, C.E., Tsesis, I., Eds.; Springer International Publishing: Cham, Switzerland, 2017; pp. 39–60.
20. Yilmaz, S.; Kuru, B.; Altuna-Kirac, E. Enamel matrix proteins in the treatment of periodontal sites with horizontal type of bone loss. *J. Clin. Periodontol.* **2003**, *30*, 197–206. [CrossRef] [PubMed]
21. Nemcovsky, C.E.; Zahavi, S.; Moses, O.; Kebudi, E.; Artzi, Z.; Beny, L.; Weinreb, M. Effect of enamel matrix protein derivative on healing of surgical supra-infrabony periodontal defects in the rat molar: A histomorphometric study. *J. Periodontol.* **2006**, *77*, 996–1002. [CrossRef] [PubMed]

22. Maymon-Gil, T.; Weinberg, E.; Nemcovsky, C.; Weinreb, M. Enamel matrix derivative promotes healing of a surgical wound in the rat oral mucosa. *J. Periodontol.* **2016**, *87*, 601–609. [CrossRef] [PubMed]
23. Tonetti, M.S.; Cortellini, P.; Lang, N.P.; Suvan, J.E.; Adriaens, P.; Dubravec, D.; Fonzar, A.; Fourmousis, I.; Rasperini, G.; Rossi, R.; et al. Clinical outcomes following treatment of human intrabony defects with gtr/bone replacement material or access flap alone. A multicenter randomized controlled clinical trial. *J. Clin. Periodontol.* **2004**, *31*, 770–776. [CrossRef] [PubMed]
24. Keila, S.; Nemcovsky, C.E.; Moses, O.; Artzi, Z.; Weinreb, M. In vitro effects of enamel matrix proteins on rat bone marrow cells and gingival fibroblasts. *J. Dent. Res.* **2004**, *83*, 134–138. [CrossRef] [PubMed]
25. Zeldich, E.; Koren, R.; Nemcovsky, C.; Weinreb, M. Enamel matrix derivative stimulates human gingival fibroblast proliferation via erk. *J. Dent. Res.* **2007**, *86*, 41–46. [CrossRef] [PubMed]
26. Zeldich, E.; Koren, R.; Dard, M.; Nemcovsky, C.; Weinreb, M. Egfr in enamel matrix derivative-induced gingival fibroblast mitogenesis. *J. Dent. Res.* **2008**, *87*, 850–855. [CrossRef] [PubMed]
27. Weinberg, E.; Zeldich, E.; Weinreb, M.M.; Moses, O.; Nemcovsky, C.; Weinreb, M. Prostaglandin e2 inhibits the proliferation of human gingival fibroblasts via the ep2 receptor and epac. *J. Cell. Biochem.* **2009**, *108*, 207–215. [CrossRef] [PubMed]
28. Zeldich, E.; Koren, R.; Dard, M.; Weinberg, E.; Weinreb, M.; Nemcovsky, C.E. Enamel matrix derivative induces the expression of tissue inhibitor of matrix metalloproteinase-3 in human gingival fibroblasts via extracellular signal-regulated kinase. *J. Periodontal Res.* **2010**, *45*, 200–206. [CrossRef] [PubMed]
29. Weinberg, E.; Topaz, M.; Dard, M.; Lyngstadaas, P.; Nemcovsky, C.; Weinreb, M. Differential effects of prostaglandin e(2) and enamel matrix derivative on the proliferation of human gingival and dermal fibroblasts and gingival keratinocytes. *J. Periodontal Res.* **2010**, *45*, 731–740. [CrossRef] [PubMed]
30. Miron, R.J.; Dard, M.; Weinreb, M. Enamel matrix derivative, inflammation and soft tissue wound healing. *J. Periodontal Res.* **2015**, *50*, 555–569. [CrossRef] [PubMed]
31. Miron, R.J.; Sculean, A.; Cochran, D.L.; Froum, S.; Zucchelli, G.; Nemcovsky, C.; Donos, N.; Lyngstadaas, S.P.; Deschner, J.; Dard, M.; et al. Twenty years of enamel matrix derivative: The past, the present and the future. *J. Clin. Periodontol.* **2016**, *43*, 668–683. [CrossRef] [PubMed]
32. Bosshardt, D.D. Biological mediators and periodontal regeneration: A review of enamel matrix proteins at the cellular and molecular levels. *J. Clin. Periodontol.* **2008**, *35*, 87–105. [CrossRef] [PubMed]
33. Murphy, K.G.; Gunsolley, J.C. Guided tissue regeneration for the treatment of periodontal intrabony and furcation defects. A systematic review. *Ann. Periodontol.* **2003**, *8*, 266–302. [CrossRef] [PubMed]
34. Cortellini, P.; Tonetti, M.S. Clinical concepts for regenerative therapy in intrabony defects. *Periodontol. 2000* **2015**, *68*, 282–307. [CrossRef] [PubMed]
35. Trombelli, L.; Farina, R.; Franceschetti, G.; Calura, G. Single-flap approach with buccal access in periodontal reconstructive procedures. *J. Periodontol.* **2009**, *80*, 353–360. [CrossRef] [PubMed]
36. Trombelli, L.; Simonelli, A.; Pramstraller, M.; Wikesjo, U.M.; Farina, R. Single flap approach with and without guided tissue regeneration and a hydroxyapatite biomaterial in the management of intraosseous periodontal defects. *J. Periodontol.* **2010**, *81*, 1256–1263. [CrossRef] [PubMed]
37. Trombelli, L.; Simonelli, A.; Schincaglia, G.P.; Cucchi, A.; Farina, R. Single-flap approach for surgical debridement of deep intraosseous defects: A randomized controlled trial. *J. Periodontol.* **2012**, *83*, 27–35. [CrossRef] [PubMed]
38. Farina, R.; Simonelli, A.; Minenna, L.; Rasperini, G.; Trombelli, L. Single-flap approach in combination with enamel matrix derivative in the treatment of periodontal intraosseous defects. *Int. J. Periodontics Restor. Dent.* **2014**, *34*, 497–506. [CrossRef] [PubMed]
39. Farina, R.; Simonelli, A.; Rizzi, A.; Pramstraller, M.; Cucchi, A.; Trombelli, L. Early postoperative healing following buccal single flap approach to access intraosseous periodontal defects. *Clin. Oral Investig.* **2013**, *17*, 1573–1583. [CrossRef] [PubMed]
40. Schincaglia, G.P.; Hebert, E.; Farina, R.; Simonelli, A.; Trombelli, L. Single versus double flap approach in periodontal regenerative treatment. *J. Clin. Periodontol.* **2015**, *42*, 557–566. [CrossRef] [PubMed]
41. Farina, R.; Simonelli, A.; Minenna, L.; Rasperini, G.; Schincaglia, G.P.; Tomasi, C.; Trombelli, L. Change in the gingival margin profile after the single flap approach in periodontal intraosseous defects. *J. Periodontol.* **2015**, *86*, 1038–1046. [CrossRef] [PubMed]
42. Trombelli, L.; Farina, R. Clinical outcomes with bioactive agents alone or in combination with grafting or guided tissue regeneration. *J. Clin. Periodontol.* **2008**, *35*, 117–135. [CrossRef] [PubMed]

43. Tu, Y.K.; Needleman, I.; Chambrone, L.; Lu, H.K.; Faggion, C.M., Jr. A bayesian network meta-analysis on comparisons of enamel matrix derivatives, guided tissue regeneration and their combination therapies. *J. Clin. Periodontol.* **2012**, *39*, 303–314. [CrossRef] [PubMed]
44. Matarasso, M.; Iorio-Siciliano, V.; Blasi, A.; Ramaglia, L.; Salvi, G.E.; Sculean, A. Enamel matrix derivative and bone grafts for periodontal regeneration of intrabony defects. A systematic review and meta-analysis. *Clin. Oral Investig.* **2015**, *19*, 1581–1593. [CrossRef] [PubMed]
45. Sato, S.; Yamada, K.; Kato, T.; Haryu, K.; Ito, K. Treatment of miller class III recessions with enamel matrix derivative (emdogain) in combination with subepithelial connective tissue grafting. *Int. J. Periodontics Restor. Dent.* **2006**, *26*, 71–77.
46. Carnio, J.; Camargo, P.M.; Kenney, E.B.; Schenk, R.K. Histological evaluation of 4 cases of root coverage following a connective tissue graft combined with an enamel matrix derivative preparation. *J. Periodontol.* **2002**, *73*, 1534–1543. [CrossRef] [PubMed]
47. Rasperini, G.; Silvestri, M.; Schenk, R.K.; Nevins, M.L. Clinical and histologic evaluation of human gingival recession treated with a subepithelial connective tissue graft and enamel matrix derivative (emdogain): A case report. *Int. J. Periodontics Restor. Dent.* **2000**, *20*, 269–275.
48. Zucchelli, G.; Mazzotti, C.; Tirone, F.; Mele, M.; Bellone, P.; Mounssif, I. The connective tissue graft wall technique and enamel matrix derivative to improve root coverage and clinical attachment levels in miller class IV gingival recession. *Int. J. Periodontics Restor. Dent.* **2014**, *34*, 601–609. [CrossRef]
49. Trombelli, L.; Simonelli, A.; Minenna, L.; Rasperini, G.; Farina, R. Effect of a connective tissue graft in combination with a single flap approach in the regenerative treatment of intraosseous defects. *J. Periodontol.* **2017**, *88*, 348–356. [CrossRef] [PubMed]
50. Cortellini, P.; Tonetti, M.S. Minimally invasive surgical technique and enamel matrix derivative in intra-bony defects. I: Clinical outcomes and morbidity. *J. Clin. Periodontol.* **2007**, *34*, 1082–1088. [CrossRef] [PubMed]

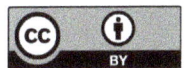

© 2018 by the authors. Licensee MDPI, Basel, Switzerland. This article is an open access article distributed under the terms and conditions of the Creative Commons Attribution (CC BY) license (http://creativecommons.org/licenses/by/4.0/).

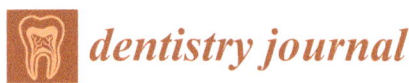

Review

Regeneration of the Periodontal Apparatus in Aggressive Periodontitis Patients

Zvi Artzi *, Shiran Sudri, Ori Platner and Avital Kozlovsky

Department of Periodontology and Oral Implantology, Tel Aviv University, Tel Aviv-Yafo 69979, Israel; sudri.shiran@gmail.com (S.S.); ori.platner@gmail.com (O.P.); kavital@tauex.tau.ac.il (A.K.)
* Correspondence: zviartzi@tauex.tau.ac.il

Received: 27 December 2018; Accepted: 22 February 2019; Published: 8 March 2019

Abstract: The purpose of this study is to evaluate and compare, retrospectively, the outcome of two different periodontal regeneration procedures in patients suffering from aggressive periodontitis (AgP). Twenty-eight patients were diagnosed with AgP, suffering from several intra-bony defects (IBD); that were treated by one of two periodontal regeneration techniques randomly assigned to each patient: a. guided tissue regeneration (GTR) or b. an application of extracted enamel matrix derivatives (EMD) combined with demineralized bone xenograft particles (DBX). Probing pocket depth (PPD), clinical attachment level (CAL), and gingival recession were recorded. Pre-treatment and follow-up (up to 10 years from the surgery) recordings were analyzed statistically within and between groups. A significant reduction was shown at time on PPD and CAL values, however, not between subject groups. CAL values decreased in all sites. At the EMD group (44 sites), CAL gain was 1.92 mm ($\pm$1.68) from pre-treatment to follow-up (p < 0.001) and at the GTR group (12 sites) CAL gain of 2.27 ($\pm$1.82) mm. In conclusion, 1–10 years observations have shown that surgical treatment of AgP patients by either GTR or by application of EMD/DBX results in similar successful clinical results.

Keywords: periodontal regeneration; aggressive periodontitis; deproteinized bovine bone; enamel matrix derivatives (Emdogain®); guided tissue regeneration (GTR)

---

1. Introduction

Aggressive periodontitis (AgP) is a periodontal disease characterized by a rapid loss of periodontal tissue. Several features describe AgP, such as early onset, involvement of a few or multiple teeth, and a relatively rapid progression [1,2]. There are two distinguishable patterns available: the localized form that involves the first molars and the incisors and up to two additional teeth, and the generalized form with an extensive destructive pattern [2–5]. Recently [6], the classification of the periodontal entities has been updated to stages (I–IV) and grades (A–C). The stages are based on periodontal breakdown severity, management complexity, and the extent of the disease. Grade definitions are based on the progression which in principal is related to risk factors. Practically, most of the AgP cases would be classified as stage III grade B or C.

There is a consensus that the main contributing factors are related to an impaired immune response [7], host-environment interactions and intra-host gene [1,8], and there is ethnic attribution whereas AgP is more frequent in certain geographic regions [9].

The therapy goal of AgP is to completely prevent and stop the progression of the disease, to maintain health and to regenerate the lost deprived periodontium; these goals are similar to those of chronic adult periodontitis [2]. Systematic reviews [10,11] claimed that the mechanical therapy may be as effective as the other one in both conditions.

Two different approaches may accomplish regenerative periodontal therapy: a. guided tissue regeneration (GTR) by selective cell population using tissue barriers [12] or b. enamel matrix derivates (EMD) application of tissue morphogenic factors to promote tissue growth [13,14].

Some clinical trials were performed in order to test the combined EMD/demineralized bone xenograft particles (DBX) in the belief that it may have certain qualities of a bioactive bone substitute [15–27]. On the other hand, previous studies that used critical size defect in rats failed to support these claims [28–30]. Also, in meta-analyses [31–33], it was not proven that there is a significant contribution of this combination. However, in 2012 Miron et al. have shown that EMD enhance osteoblast and PDL cell proliferation, differentiation and attachment to DBX particles in vitro. In vivo recent data [34] has shown that the combination between EMD and DBX particles has the ability to enhance and accelerate new bone formation in rat osseous defects.

Many randomized trials have shown encouraging results of periodontal therapy in Chronic periodontitis (ChP) patients, however, there are only a few reports that claim clinical success using either the GTR technique in AgP patients [35–37] or the EMD application [38–41]. Moreover, most of these reports, especially those related to the later, are based on small group of patients with no clinical standardization and/or follow-up protocols.

The aim of this this study is to retrospectively evaluate the efficacy via one of the surgical regenerative options, GTR or EMD w/wo biomaterial filler, among AgP patients in 1–10 years follow-up.

2. Periodontal Regeneration Procedures

2.1. Guided Tissue Regeneration (GTR) Procedure

Prior to surgery, patients were admitted to rinse their mouth with 0.2% chlorohexidine, followed by local anesthesia, buccal and lingual infiltration. Muco-periosteal flaps were reflected in order to expose widely the intra-bony defects, while using the papillary preservation technique (PPT) described by Takei et al. [42,43] and Cortellini et al. [44]. in order to preserve the interproximal soft tissue. Horizontal interproximal incision was performed on the opposite side (buccal or lingual) considering the site with the deepest probing pocket depth (PPD) value. Root planning and soft tissue debridement was conducted to smooth the exposed root surface.

A sample simulated matrix was trimmed to prepare a customized fit resorbable collagen membrane (Figures 1 and 2, case #4). DBX particles (500–1000 µ) were placed to fill the intra bony defect, followed by coverage with the trimmed membrane. Primary soft tissue closure was achieved by releasing the flaps and stabilizing it, executing interrupted internal mattress sutures to achieve complete closure in the interproximal areas [45]. (Figures 1 and 2)

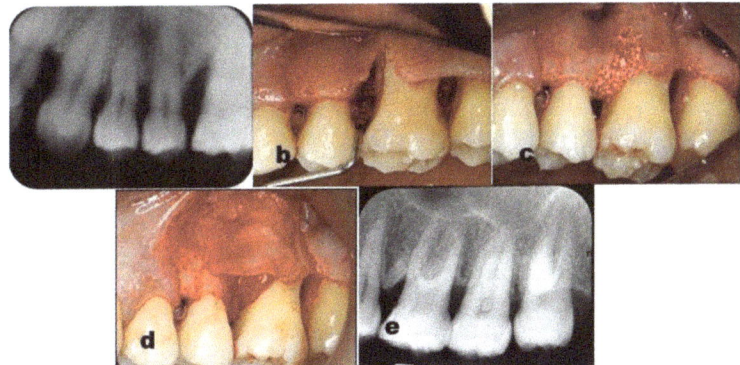

Figure 1. Case # 4 of the guided tissue regeneration (GTR) group, upper left sextant. The pre surgery periapical radiograph (**a**) demonstrates an extensive periodontal destruction around on the mesial aspect of the first molar. (**b**) The periodontal probe shows a 2-wall intrabony component of 7mm, which was filled by bovine bone mineral particles (**c**) and covered by a collagen membrane (**d**). two years follow-up periapical radiograph (**e**) shows bone filling around on the first molar.

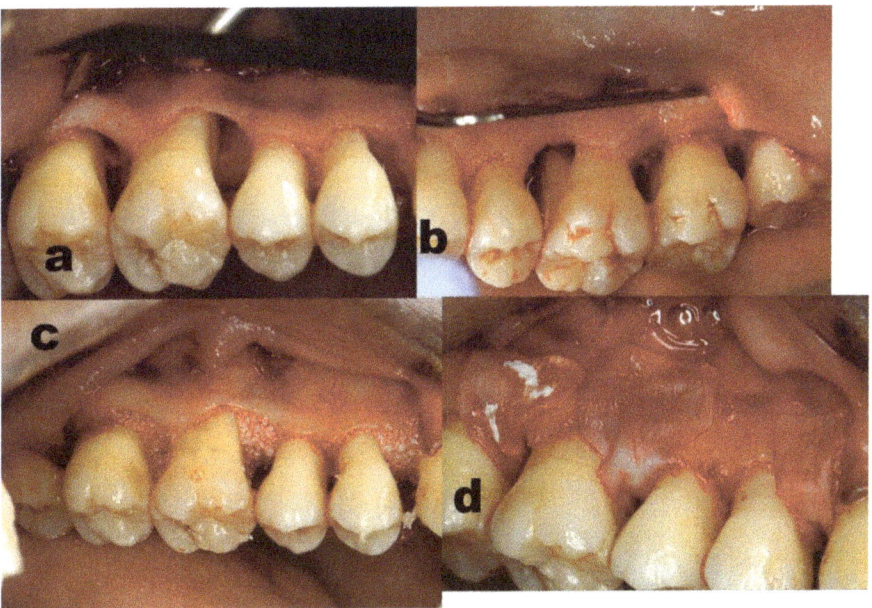

Figure 2. Case # 4 of the GTR group, upper right sextant. (**a,b**) Buccal and palatal view of the crestal bone topography. BBM particles inserted to fill the defects (**c**) followed by overlay resorbable collagen membranes (**d**).

2.2. Periodontal Regeneration by Application of Enamel Matrix Derivatives (EMD)

Prior to surgery, patients were admitted to rinse their mouth with 0.2% chlorohexidine, followed by local anesthesia, buccal and lingual infiltration. Muco-periosteal flaps were reflected in order to expose widely the intra-bony defects, while using the PPT described by Takei et al. [42,43] and Cortellini et al. [44] in order to preserve the interproximal soft tissue. Horizontal interproximal incision was performed on the opposite side (buccal or lingual) considering the site with the deepest PPD value. Root planning and soft tissue debridement was conducted to smooth the exposed root surface.

The exposed roots were conditioned with 24% EDTA for 2 minutes, followed by saline rinsing, and by applying EMD gel (Emdogain®) (Figures 3 and 4, Case #2). Avoiding bleeding in these sites was executed. In some cases, DBX soaked in EMD gel were then added to fill the defect. Full soft tissue closure was obtained by releasing the flaps and stabilizing it, executing interrupted internal mattress sutures to achieve complete closure in the interproximal areas [45].

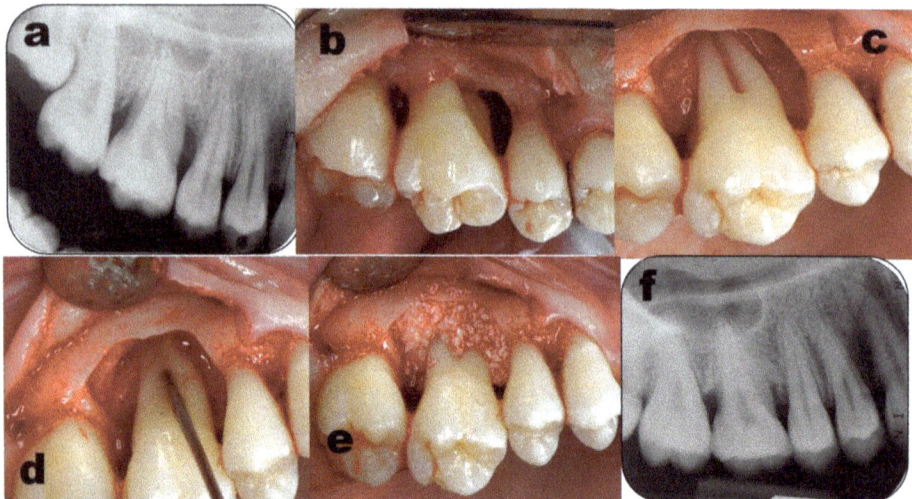

Figure 3. Case # 2 of the enamel matrix derivatives (EMD) group, upper right sextant. Pre surgery periapical radiograph (**a**) shows an extensive periodontal destruction around on the distal aspect of the first molar. Buccal (**b**) and palatal (**c**) aspects of the debrided roots. EMD gel was applied along the exposed roots (**d**) followed by BBM particles as a bio-material filler (**e**). four years follow-up periapical radiograph (**f**) shows bone filling around the first molar.

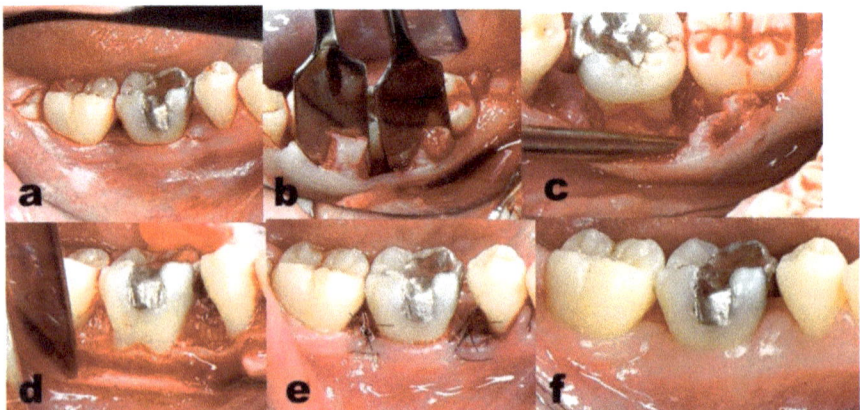

Figure 4. Case # 2 of the EMD group, lower right sextant. Papillary preserve technique flap elevation technique (**a**,**b**) performed to exposed the periodontal defect (**c**). EMD gel was applied on the debrided roots followed by BBM particles (**d**). In order to obtain full soft tissue closure the flaps were sutured (**e**). At 1 month, immaculate healing was evident (**f**). In order to achieve full closure, note the preservation performed of the interproximal col tissue (**b**), subsequently.

Strict post-op instructions were given to candidates from both groups. At 2 weeks, sutures were removed. Patients were instructed to gently clean the site with gauze soaked in CHX solution. During the maintenance phase, for the first month, patients were monitored weekly, followed by monthly visits for half a year, and once every three months later. Recall visits focused on reinforcement of oral hygiene performance and supra-gingival prophylactic cleaning. PPD, clinical attachment level (CAL) and recession height (Rec) were recorded at 6, 12, month post-surgery. Peri-apical and bite-wings radiographs were taken at the initial examination and after 6 and 12 months (Figures 3–5).

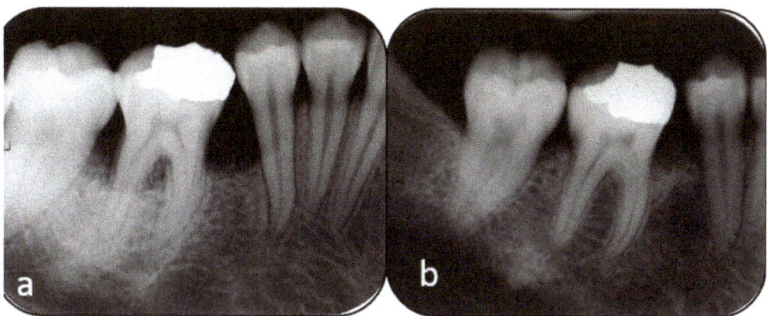

Figure 5. The pre (**a**) and post (**b**) periapical radiographs of Case #2 of the EMD group, lower right first molar. Note the bone filling on the mesial and distal aspect of the lower right first molar.

2.3. Materials and Methods

Tel Aviv University ethics committee approved this study; 28 young (15–39 years old) healthy patients 12 males and 16 females that were diagnosed with AgP randomly selected; 6 patients (12 surgical sites) were treated by the GTR method, and therefore called the GTR group; 12 patients (54 surgical sites) were treated by the EMD method, and therefore called the EMD group.

The first appointment included extra and intra oral examinations including, a thorough periodontal chart, full mouth peri-apical radiographs and study models.

PPD, CAL, and the height of exposed roots (Rec) were recorded in all destroyed sites. As performed in previous study (Artzi et al.) [46], at each periodontally involved interproximal/inter-radicular intra-bony site, the deepest probing depth was recorded. Mean PPD and CAL (Tables 1 and 2) represent the execution of the average measurements of all sites of each treated intra-bony defects (IBD) in each patient. For example, in a given interproximal IBD, mean probing depth was calculated as the average of the disto-buccal, disto-lingual/palatal of the mesial root (tooth) surface and the mesio-buccal and mesio-lingual/palatal of the distal root (tooth) surface. Therefore, each mean PPD site represents only the involved IBD without the neighboring unaffected shallow ones. Horizontal furcation involvement was assessed, in the inter-radicular areas [47]. The plaque score index (PI) [48] and bleeding on probing (BOP) [49] were monitored carefully. During each re-evaluation visit these parameters were repeated.

In the pre-surgical phase, the patients went through a meticulous non-surgical therapy including OHI and motivation, full mouth scaling and root debridement in conjunction followed by adjunctive systemic antibiotics of Amoxicillin 500 mg + metronidazole 250 mg (TID) for a week [50–52].

Table 1. GTR group, pre-op and follow-up periodontal probing pocket depth (PPD) mean measurements.

Site	PPD pre	CAL pre	PPD curr	CAL curr	PDR [1]	CAL GAIN
1	5.5	5.5	5	5	0.5	0.5
2	6.5	7	3.5	4.25	3	2.75
3	4	4	2	2	2	2
4	5.5	5.5	5.5	5.5	0	0
5	4.5	4.5	5.25	5.5	−0.75	−1
6	7	7.5	4.75	4.75	2.25	2.75
7	6.5	6.5	3.5	3.5	3	3
8	6	6	3.75	3.75	2.25	2.25
9	7.5	8	2.75	2.75	4.75	5.25
10	8.5	8.75	3	3.25	5.5	5.5
11	7.5	7.5	3.5	5	4	2.5
12	5.75	5.75	4	4	1.75	1.75
Average [2]	6.23	6.37	3.87	4.10	2.36	2.27
SD	1.24	1.37	1.02	1.06	1.79	1.82

[1] PDR—probing depth reduction. [2] The average of 4 probing depth measurements at the disto-buccal, mesio-buccal, mesio-lingual and disto-lingual of each given intra-bony defects (IBD) site.

Table 2. EMD group, pre-op and follow-up periodontal probing pocket depth (PPD) mean measurements.

site	PPD pre	CAL pre	PPD curr	CAL curr	PDR [1]	CAL GAIN
1	5	5.5	3	3.5	2	2
2	4.75	5.75	2.25	3.75	2.5	2
3	3.75	3.75	3	3.75	0.75	0
4	7	7	2.75	3.75	4.25	3.25
5	4	4	4.5	4.5	−0.5	−0.5
6	6.5	6.5	4.25	4.25	2.25	2.25
7	4.5	4.5	3.75	3.75	0.75	0.75
8	5.5	5.5	6.5	6.5	−1	−1
9	5.5	5.5	3.75	3.75	1.75	1.75
10	5	5	3	3	2	2
11	6	6.75	6	6.75	0	0
12	8	8	6.5	7.25	1.5	0.75
13	7	7	3.25	4.5	3.75	2.5
14	6.5	9	2	4	4.5	5
15	5	6.5	4	6	1	0.5
16	7.5	10.25	3.25	5.75	4.25	4.5
17	4.5	6	3.25	4.25	1.25	1.75
18	5.75	5.75	2.25	2.25	3.5	3.5
19	5	5	3.5	3.5	1.5	1.5
20	7.5	8	6	6	1.5	2
21	4.5	5	4.5	4.5	0	0.5
22	7.5	7.5	3	4	4.5	3.5
23	3.5	5.25	2	3.25	1.5	2
24	5.5	5.5	7	7	1.5	−1.5
25	6.5	7	6.25	6.75	0.25	0.25
26	4	4.5	2.5	4	1.5	0.5
27	4.5	5	3.5	3.5	1	1.5
27	5.25	7.25	2.5	3.5	2.75	3.75

Table 2. Cont.

site	PPD pre	CAL pre	PPD curr	CAL curr	PDR [1]	CAL GAIN
29	4	6.5	3	5.25	1	1.25
30	4.75	6	2	2.5	2.75	3.5
31	7	8	3.25	3.75	3.75	4.25
32	4.75	4.75	3.25	4.25	1.5	0.5
33	6	6	3.5	4.5	2.5	1.5
34	6.75	7.5	4.75	5.75	2	1.75
35	6.25	7.25	5.25	5.75	1	1.5
36	6.75	6.75	4	4	2.75	2.75
37	6.75	6.75	4	4	2.75	2.75
38	6.5	6.75	7	7	−0.5	−0.25
39	5.5	6	extracted			
40	8.75	9	3	3	5.75	6
41	8.5	8.75	3	3	5.5	5.75
42	3.75	3.75	2	3	1.75	0.75
43	6	6	2	3	4	3
44	4.75	5	2.25	2.75	2.5	2.25
45	5.5	6.5	2	2.5	3.5	4
46	7	9	3.25	4.25	3.75	4.75
47	4	5.75	5.25	5.75	−1.25	0
48	4.25	4.25	3	3.5	1.25	0.75
49	4	5	2.75	3.75	1.25	1.25
50	4.25	4.25	3.5	3.5	0.75	0.75
51	4	4	3.25	3.25	0.75	0.75
52	3.5	3.5	2.75	2.75	0.75	0.75
53	5.75	5.75	3	3.25	2.75	2.5
54	7	7.75	3.75	3.75	3.25	4
Average [2]	5.58	6.16	3.64	4.24	1.94	1.92
SD	1.34	1.52	1.35	1.3	1.64	1.68

[1] PDR—probing depth reduction. [2] The average of 4 probing depth measurements at the disto-buccal, mesio-buccal, mesio-lingual and disto-lingual of each given IBD site.

3. Results

Considering the strict oral hygiene maintenance program, patient compliance was very satisfactory. No adverse effects were noted throughout either mode of treatment. In 3 patients, a distinctive familial inheritance along their family tree was noted. However, they responded to treatment immaculately.

Periodontal indices were re-measured, upon re-evaluation of the non-surgical phase. Practically, a clinical improvement was evident as related to the periodontal indices. Tables 1 and 2 show PPD reduction and CAL gain at follow-up, up to 10 years post the completion of the surgical phase. Since there was no significant approval on the PPD and CAL indices at the extensive IBD sites, the baseline clinical and follow-up, 10-year recordings of CAL indices are listed in the Tables.

Follow up (up to 10 years) PPD in the GTR group (n = 6; sites = 12) was reduced from 6.23 mm (±1.24 standard deviation (SD)) to 3.875 mm (±1.02). Mean PPD reduction was 2.35 mm ($p < 0.001$). Mean CAL in the GTR group reduced from 6.375 (±1.37) to 4.1 mm (±1.06); mean CAL gain was 2.27 mm ($p < 0.001$).

In the EMD group (n = 22; sites = 54), mean PPD reduced from 5.58 mm (±1.34) to 3.64 mm (±1.36). Mean reduction was 1.95 mm ($p < 0.001$). Mean CAL was reduced from 6.16 mm (±1.52) to 4.26) mm (±1.3); mean CAL gain of 1.92 mm ($p < 0.001$). Within each group, PPD reduction and CAL gain between the measurements were statistically significant.

However, tests of between subjects (GTR and EMD) effects, showed no statistical difference in regard to PPD ($p > 0.005$) nor to CAL ($p > 0.005$).

4. Discussion

There are two different methods to support periodontal regeneration: guided tissue regeneration (GTR) principles, and amelogenin-derived protein i.e., EMD root-surface soaking. In spite of the distinctive biological activity differences between the two methods, similar outcomes were achieved by both modalities in 1–10 years follow-up.

In the current study, GTR treated sites presented PPD reduction of 37.7% and CAL gain of 35.6%. EMD sites showed similar results with PPD reduction of 34.9% and CAL gain of 31.2%. Follow-up radiographs supported the clinical measurements, showing consistent bone augmentation and re-formation of periodontal ligament space and lamina dura (Figure 1, Figure 3 and Figure 5).

Regeneration capacity is effected well by the IBD morphology. Thus, other shortcomings of the study design could be the fact that different IBD morphology were not considered as a significant variable factor in the interpretation of the outcome where they should be.

In order to achieve successful healing several indications are required; wound stability, re-vascularization, and the establishment of complete soft tissue closure; in regenerative treatment these are mandatory prerequisites for successful results. Furthely, flap management via PPT should enhance the outcome of regenerative procedures [45,53]. For these reasons we used those clinical measures in both groups.

It seems that in addition to meticulous surgical execution, strict maintenance and patient compliance are key factors, regardless the surgical mode of operation.

As specified, AgP is a rapidly progressing inflammatory disease. However, devoted care may result in quite predictable long term success [11,37].

ChP and AgP have shown distinctive different etiological/contributing factors, where the later one shows an accelerated mode of aggressiveness and rapid destructiom [1]. As a consequence, the effectiveness of regenerative periodontal treatment of intrabony defects in AgP, would be of utmost importance to maintain a successful long term periodontal heaelth

It has been claimed that in severe chronic periodontitis GTR and EMD result in periodontal restitution [12,54–73]. Surprisingly, there is not enough data available regarding AgP [74,75]. However, some studies claim for successful results using either GTR procedures [35] or EMD application [36]. Enamel matrix proteins in cases of ChP seems to support wound healing and new periodontal tissue formation in IBD sites in AgP cases as well.

One can assume that although consensus reports [76] as well as systematic reviews [71] did not differentiate between IBD treatment modality of patients diagnosed with AgP and/or ChP cases, that these sites successfully healed and maintained.

If we implicate laboratory research to our research, our findings are consistent. No statistically significant differences in immunologic and microbial parameters between subjects with AgP and ChP have been presented in several reports [77,78]. Another review performed by Deas and Mealy [10] agreed that long term outcome could be comparable with blurred boundaries in ChP and Agp.

There is no accepted statement regarding the efficacy of regenerative procedures using GTR techniques in AgP patients, although few reports examined it [35,36,75,79,80], or EMD application [39–41,74,81,82]. In the current study we pressent a long time efficacy.

Combining GTR with a biomaterial grafting material [15–23,26,83] have been extensively investigated showing that the addition of a xenograft such as DBX resulted in encouraging results in IBD in ChP. Thus, this would be related to the excellent biomaterial biocompatible and conductive properties rather than to the unproven induction as shown earlier [28–30].

In a Cochrane systematic review, Esposito et al. [71], stated that there was no clinically significant differences between GTR and EMD in periodontal intra-bony lesions. However, it was found that the use of bone substitute materials procedures were less associated with soft tissue marginal recession compared with the application of EMD solely.

Practically, there is great significance of adding the biomaterial scaffold (DBX) whether in the GTR and/or EMD technique in order to provide maintenance of the volume of the filled defect [84]) and thus, enhance the clinical outcome.

In the EMD group, no selective barrier was used, and it can be assumed that the added biomaterial particles gave mechanical support to the soft tissue over-lay during the healing phase.

Supporting our previous study (Artzi et al.) [46] both therapy modalities are proven to achieve comparable clinical outcome i.e., stability of the soft tissue position, minimal recession and ease the ability of plaque control performance.

In conclusion, among AgP patients successful regenerative approach treatment can be achieved in a predictable manner. Whereas, the key seems to be the meticulous treatment mode for both techniques followed by strict supportive periodontal maintenance.

5. Conclusions

The two approaches of periodontal regeneration, guided tissue regeneration (GTR) w/wo DBX and the application of enamel matrix derivatives (EMD) w/wo DBX, achieve comparable clinical outcomes.

Successful regenerative approach treatment can be achieved predictably in aggressive periodontitis patients. The key seems to be the meticulous surgical treatment approach and a careful soft tissue flap management, for both techniques followed by a strict supportive periodontal maintenance.

Author Contributions: Conceptualization, Z.A. and S.S; Methodology, Z.A. and S.S.; Validation, Z.A. and S.S, K.A., O.P. and Z.Z.; Formal Analysis, Z.A. and S.S.; Investigation Z.A. and S.S; Resources Z.A. and S.S, K.A., O.P.; Data Curation, Z.A., S.S., K.A., O.P.; Writing-Original Draft Preparation, Z.A. and S.S.; Writing-Review & Editing, Z.A. and S.S.; Visualization, Z.A., S.S., K.A. and O.P.; Supervision, Z.A., S.S., K.A., O.P.; Project Administration, Z.A., S.S, K.A., O.P.; Funding Acquisition, Z.A., S.S., K.A., O.P.

Funding: This research received no external funding

Conflicts of Interest: The authors declare no conflict of interest

References

1. Albandar, J.M. Aggressive periodontitis: Case definition and diagnostic criteria. *Periodontology* 2000, 65, 13–26. [CrossRef] [PubMed]
2. Armitage, G.C. Development of a classification system for periodontal diseases and conditions. *Ann. Periodontol.* **1999**, 4, 1–6. [CrossRef] [PubMed]
3. Baer, P.N. The case for periodontosis as a clinical entity. *J. Periodontol.* **1971**, 42, 516–520. [CrossRef] [PubMed]
4. Baer, P.N.; Socransky, S.S. Periodontosis: Case report with long-term follow-up. *Periodontal Case Rep.* **1979**, 1, 1–6. [PubMed]
5. Hørmand, J.; Frandsen, A. Juvenile periodontitis. Localization of bone loss in relation to age, sex, and teeth. *J. Clin. Periodontol.* **1979**, 6, 407–416. [CrossRef] [PubMed]
6. Tonetti, M.S.; Greenwell, H.; Kornman, K.S. Staging and grading of periodontitis: Framework and proposal of a new classification and case definition. *J. Clin. Periodontol.* **2018**, 45 (Suppl. 20), S149–S161. [CrossRef] [PubMed]
7. Khocht, A.; Albandar, J.M. Aggressive forms of periodontitis secondary to systemic disorders. *Periodontology* 2000, 65, 134–148. [CrossRef] [PubMed]
8. Vieira, A.R.; Albandar, J.M. Role of genetic factors in the pathogenesis of aggressive periodontitis. *Periodontology* 2000, 65, 92–106. [CrossRef] [PubMed]
9. Susin, C.; Haas, A.N.; Albandar, J.M. Epidemiology and demographics of aggressive periodontitis. *Periodontology* 2000, 65, 27–45. [CrossRef] [PubMed]
10. Deas, D.E.; Mealey, B.L. Response of chronic and aggressive periodontitis to treatment. *Periodontology* 2000, 53, 154–166. [CrossRef] [PubMed]
11. Nibali, L.; Farias, B.C.; Vajgel, A.; Tu, Y.K.; Donos, N. Tooth loss in aggressive periodontitis: A systematic review. *J. Dent. Res.* **2013**, 92, 868–875. [CrossRef] [PubMed]

12. Gottlow, J.; Nyman, S.; Lindhe, J.; Karring, T.; Wennström, J. New attachment formation in the human periodontium by guided tissue regeneration. Case reports. *J. Clin. Periodontol.* **1986**, *13*, 604–616. [CrossRef] [PubMed]
13. Hammarström, L. Enamel matrix, cementum development and regeneration. *J. Clin. Periodontol.* **1997**, *24*, 658–668. [CrossRef]
14. Heijl, L.; Heden, G.; Svärdström, G.; Ostgren, A. Enamel matrix derivative (EMDOGAIN) in the treatment of intrabony periodontal defects. *J. Clin. Periodontol.* **1997**, *24*, 705–714. [CrossRef] [PubMed]
15. Lekovic, V.; Camargo, P.M.; Weinlaender, M.; Nedic, M.; Aleksic, Z.; Kenney, E.B. A comparison between enamel matrix proteins used alone or in combination with bovine porousbone mineral in the treatment of intrabony periodontal defects in humans. *J. Periodontol.* **2000**, *71*, 1110–1116. [CrossRef] [PubMed]
16. Lekovic, V.; Camargo, P.M.; Weinlaender, M.; Kenney, E.B.; Vasilic, N. Combination use of bovine porous bone mineral, enamel matrix proteins, and a bioabsorbable membrane in intrabony periodontal defects in humans. *J. Periodontol.* **2001**, *72*, 583–589. [CrossRef] [PubMed]
17. Camargo, P.M.; Lekovic, V.; Weinlaender, M.; Vasilic, N.; Kenney, E.B.; Madzarevic, M. The effectiveness of enamel matrix proteins used in combination with bovine porous bone mineral in the treatment of intrabony defects in humans. *J. Clin. Periodontol.* **2001**, *28*, 1016–1022. [CrossRef] [PubMed]
18. Scheyer, E.T.; Velasquez-Plata, D.; Brunsvold, M.A.; Lasho, D.J.; Mellonig, J.T. A clinical comparison of a bovine-derived xenograft used alone and in combination with enamel matrix derivative for the treatment of periodontal osseous defects in humans. *J. Periodontol.* **2002**, *73*, 423–432. [CrossRef] [PubMed]
19. Velasquez-Plata, D.; Scheyer, E.T.; Mellonig, J.T. Clinical comparison of an enamel matrix derivative used alone or in combination with a bovine-derived xenograft for the treatment of periodontal osseous defects in humans. *J. Periodontol.* **2002**, *73*, 433–440. [CrossRef] [PubMed]
20. Sculean, A.; Chiantella, G.C.; Windisch, P.; Gera, I.; Reich, E. Clinical evaluation of an enamel matrix protein derivative (Emdogain) combined with a bovine-derived xenograft (Bio-Oss) for the treatment of intrabony periodontal defects in humans. *Int. J. Periodontics Restor. Dent.* **2002**, *22*, 259–267.
21. Sculean, A.; Windisch, P.; Keglevich, T.; Chiantella, G.C.; Gera, I.; Donos, N. Clinical and histologic evaluation of human intrabony defects treated with an enamel matrix protein derivative combined with a bovine-derived xenograft. *Int. J. Periodontics Restor. Dent.* **2003**, *23*, 47–55.
22. Sculean, A.; Pietruska, M.; Schwarz, F.; Willershausen, B.; Arweiler, N.B.; Auschill, T.M. Healing of human intrabony defects following regenerative periodontal therapy with an enamel matrix protein derivative alone or combined with a bioactive glass. A controlled clinical study. *J. Clin. Periodontol.* **2005**, *32*, 111–117. [CrossRef] [PubMed]
23. Sculean, A.; Chiantella, G.C.; Arweiler, N.B.; Becker, J.; Schwarz, F.; Stavropoulos, A. Five-year clinical and histologic results following treatment of human intrabony defects with an enamel matrix derivative combined with a natural bone mineral. *Int. J. Periodontics Restor. Dent.* **2008**, *28*, 153–161.
24. Zucchelli, G.; Amore, C.; Montebugnoli, L.; De Sanctis, M. Enamel matrix proteins and bovine porous bone mineral in the treatment of intrabony defects: A comparative controlled clinical trial. *J. Periodontol.* **2003**, *74*, 1725–1735. [CrossRef] [PubMed]
25. Yamamoto, S.; Masuda, H.; Shibukawa, Y.; Yamada, S. Combination of bovine-derived xenografts and enamel matrix derivative in the treatment of intrabony periodontal defects in dogs. *Int. J. Periodontics Restor. Dent.* **2007**, *27*, 471–479.
26. Iorio-Siciliano, V.; Andreuccetti, G.; Blasi, A.; Matarasso, M.; Sculean, A.; Salvi, G.E. Clinical Outcomes Following Regenerative Therapy of Non-Contained Intrabony Defects Using a Deproteinized Bovine Bone Mineral Combined with Either Enamel Matrix Derivative or Collagen Membrane. *J. Periodontol.* **2014**, *85*, 1342–1350. [CrossRef] [PubMed]
27. Farina, R.; Simonelli, A.; Minenna, L.; Rasperini, G.; Trombelli, L. Single-flap approach in combination with enamel matrix derivative in the treatment of periodontal intraosseous defects. *Int. J. Periodontics Restor. Dent.* **2014**, *34*, 497–506. [CrossRef] [PubMed]
28. Donos, N.; Lang, N.P.; Karoussis, I.K.; Bosshardt, D.; Tonetti, M.; Kostopoulos, L. Effect of GBR in combination with deproteinized bovine bone mineral and/or enamel matrix proteins on the healing of critical-size defects. *Clin. Oral Implants Res.* **2004**, *15*, 101–111. [CrossRef]

29. Donos, N.; Bosshardt, D.; Lang, N.; Graziani, F.; Tonetti, M.; Karring, T.; Kostopoulos, L. Bone formation by enamel matrix proteins and xenografts: An experimental study in the rat ramus. *Clin. Oral Implants Res.* **2005**, *16*, 140–146. [CrossRef]
30. Donos, N.; Kostopoulos, L.; Tonetti, M.; Karring, T.; Lang, N.P. The effect of enamel matrix proteins and deproteinized bovine bone mineral on heterotopicbone formation. *Clin. Oral Implants Res.* **2006**, *17*, 434–438. [CrossRef]
31. Tu, Y.K.; Woolston, A.; Faggion, C.M., Jr. Do bone grafts or barrier membranes provide additional treatment effects for infrabony lesions treated with enamel matrix derivatives? A network meta-analysis of randomized-controlled trials. *J. Clin. Periodontol.* **2010**, *37*, 59–79. [CrossRef] [PubMed]
32. Verardi, S. The use of a membrane and/or a bone graft may not improve the effects of enamel matrix derivatives in infrabony defects. *J. Evid. Based Dent. Pract.* **2012**, *12*, 127–128. [CrossRef] [PubMed]
33. Miron, R.J.; Bosshardt, D.D.; Hedbom, E.; Zhang, Y.; Haenni, B.; Buser, D.; Sculean, A. Adsorption of enamel matrix proteins to a bovine-derived bone grafting material and its regulation of cell adhesion, proliferation, and differentiation. *J. Periodontol.* **2012**, *83*, 936–947. [CrossRef] [PubMed]
34. Miron, R.J.; Wei, L.; Bosshardt, D.D.; Buser, D.; Sculean, A.; Zhang, Y. Effects of enamel matrix proteins in combination with a bovine-derived natural bone mineral for the repair of bone defects. *Clin. Oral Investig.* **2014**, *18*, 471–478. [CrossRef] [PubMed]
35. Sirirat, M.; Kasetsuwan, J.; Jeffcoat, M.K. Comparison between 2 surgical techniques for the treatment of early-onset periodontitis. *J. Periodontol.* **1996**, *67*, 603–607. [CrossRef] [PubMed]
36. Zucchelli, G.; Brini, C.; de Sanctis, M. GTR treatment of intrabony defects in patients with early-onset and chronic adult periodontitis. *Int. J. Periodontics Restor. Dent.* **2002**, *22*, 323–333.
37. Buchmann, R.; Nunn, M.E.; Van Dyke, T.E.; Lange, D.E. Aggressive periodontitis: 5-year follow-up of treatment. *J. Periodontol.* **2002**, *73*, 675–683. [CrossRef] [PubMed]
38. Kiernicka, M.; Owczarek, B.; Gałkowska, E.; Wysokińska-Miszczuk, J. Use of Emdogain enamel matrix proteins in the surgical treatment of aggressive periodontitis. *Ann. Univ. Mar. Curie Sklodowska Med.* **2003**, *58*, 397–401.
39. Bonta, H.; Llambes, F.; Moretti, A.J.; Mathur, H.; Bouwsma, O.J. The use of enamel matrix protein in the treatment of localized aggressive periodontitis: A case report. *Quintessence Int.* **2003**, *34*, 247–252.
40. Miliauskaite, A.; Selimovic, D.; Hannig, M. Successful management of aggressive periodontitis by regenerative therapy (EMD): A 3-year follow-up case report. *J. Periodontol.* **2007**, *78*, 2043–2050. [CrossRef]
41. Kaner, D.; Bernimoulin, J.P.; Kleber, B.M.; Friedmann, A. Minimally invasive flap surgery and enamel matrix derivative in the treatment of localized aggressive periodontitis: Case report. *Int. J. Periodontics Restor. Dent.* **2009**, *29*, 89–97.
42. Takei, H.H.; Han, T.J.; Carranza, F.A., Jr.; Kenney, E.B.; Lekovic, V. Flap technique for periodontal bone implants. Papilla preservation technique. *J. Periodontol.* **1985**, *56*, 204–210. [CrossRef] [PubMed]
43. Takei, H.H.; Yamada, H.; Hau, T. Maxillary anterior esthetics. Preservation of the interdental papilla. *Dent. Clin. N. Am.* **1989**, *33*, 263–273. [PubMed]
44. Cortellini, P.; Prato, G.P.; Tonetti, M.S. The modified papilla preservation technique. A new surgical approach for interproximal regenerative procedures. *J. Periodontol.* **1995**, *66*, 261–266. [CrossRef] [PubMed]
45. Cortellini, P.; Tonetti, M.S.; Lang, N.P.; Suvan, J.E.; Zucchelli, G.; Vangsted, T.; Silvestri, M.; Rossi, R.; McClain, P.; Fonzar, A.; et al. The simplified papilla preservation flap in the regenerative treatment of deep intrabony defects: Clinical outcomes and postoperative morbidity. *J. Periodontol.* **2001**, *12*, 1702–1712. [CrossRef] [PubMed]
46. Artzi, Z.; Tal, H.; Platner, O.; Wasersprung, N.; Weinberg, E.; Slutzkey, S.; Gozali, N.; Carmeli, G.; Herzberg, R.; Kozlovsky, A. Deproteinized bovine bone in association with guided tissue regeneration or enamel matrix derivatives procedures in aggressive periodontitis patients: A 1-year retrospective study. *J. Clin. Periodontol.* **2015**, *42*, 547–556. [CrossRef] [PubMed]
47. Hamp, S.E.; Nyman, S.; Lindhe, J. Periodontal treatment of multirooted teeth. Results after 5 years. *J. Clin. Periodontol.* **1975**, *2*, 126–135. [CrossRef] [PubMed]
48. Turesky, S.; Gilmore, N.D.; Glickman, I. Reduced plaque formation by the chloromethyl analogue of victamine, C. *J. Periodontol.* **1970**, *41*, 41–43. [CrossRef]
49. Saxer, U.P.; Mühlemann, H.R. Motivation and education. *SSO Schweiz. Mon. Zahnheilkd.* **1975**, *85*, 905–919.

50. Van Winkelhoff, A.J.; Rodenburg, J.P.; Goené, R.J.; Abbas, F.; Winkel, E.G.; de Graaff, J. Metronidazole plus amoxicillin in the treatment of Actinobacillus actinomycetemcomitans associated periodontitis. *J. Clin. Periodontol.* **1989**, *16*, 128–131. [CrossRef]
51. Guerrero, A.; Griffiths, G.S.; Nibali, L.; Suvan, J.; Moles, D.R.; Laurell, L.; Tonetti, M.S. Adjunctive benefits of systemic amoxicillin and metronidazole in non-surgical treatment of generalized aggressive periodontitis: A randomized placebo-controlled clinical trial. *J. Clin. Periodontol.* **2005**, *32*, 1096–1107. [CrossRef] [PubMed]
52. Herrera, D.; Sanz, M.; Jepsen, S.; Needleman, I.; Roldán, S. A systematic review on the effect of systemic antimicrobials as an adjunct to scaling and root planing in periodontitis patients. *J. Clin. Periodontol.* **2002**, *29*, 136–159. [CrossRef] [PubMed]
53. Zucchelli, G.; Bernardi, F.; Montebugnoli, L.; De Sanctis, M. Enamel matrix proteins and guided tissue regeneration with titanium-reinforced expanded polytetrafluoroethylene membranes in the treatment of infrabony defects: A comparative controlled clinical trial. *J. Periodontol.* **2002**, *73*, 3–12. [CrossRef] [PubMed]
54. Sculean, A.; Donos, N.; Windisch, P.; Brecx, M.; Gera, I.; Reich, E.; Karring, T. Healing of human intrabony defects following treatment with enamel matrix proteins or guided tissue regeneration. *J. Periodontal Res.* **1999**, *34*, 310–322. [CrossRef] [PubMed]
55. Sculean, A.; Donos, N.; Blaes, A.; Lauermann, M.; Reich, E.; Brecx, M. Comparison of enamel matrix proteins and bioabsorbable membranes in the treatment of intrabony periodontal defects. A split-mouth study. *J. Periodontol.* **1999**, *70*, 255–262. [CrossRef] [PubMed]
56. Sculean, A.; Reich, E.; Chiantella, G.C.; Brecx, M. Treatment of intrabony periodontal defects with an enamel matrix protein derivative (Emdogain): A report of 32 cases. *Int. J. Periodontics Restor. Dent.* **1999**, *19*, 157–163.
57. Sculean, A.; Donos, N.; Brecx, M.; Reich, E.; Karring, T. Treatment of intrabony defects with guided tissue regeneration and enamel-matrix-proteins. An experimental study in monkeys. *J. Clin. Periodontol.* **2000**, *27*, 466–472. [CrossRef]
58. Sculean, A.; Chiantella, G.C.; Windisch, P.; Donos, N. Clinical and histologic evaluation of human intrabony defects treated with an enamel matrix protein derivative (Emdogain). *Int. J. Periodontics Restor. Dent.* **2000**, *20*, 374–381.
59. Sculean, A.; Windisch, P.; Chiantella, G.C.; Donos, N.; Brecx, M.; Reich, E. Treatment of intrabony defects with enamel matrix proteins and guided tissue regeneration. A prospective controlled clinical study. *J. Clin. Periodontol.* **2001**, *28*, 397–403. [CrossRef]
60. Sculean, A.; Donos, N.; Miliauskaite, A.; Arweiler, N.; Brecx, M. Treatment of intrabony defects with enamel matrix proteins or bioabsorbable membranes. A 4-year follow-up split-mouth study. *J. Periodontol.* **2001**, *72*, 1695–1701. [CrossRef]
61. Sculean, A.; Chiantella, G.C.; Miliauskaite, A.; Brecx, M.; Arweiler, N.B. Four-year results following treatment of intrabony periodontal defects with an enamel matrix protein derivative: A report of 46 cases. *Int. J. Periodontics Restor. Dent.* **2003**, *23*, 345–351.
62. Sculean, A.; Windisch, P.; Chiantella, G.C. Human histologic evaluation of an intrabony defect treated with enamel matrix derivative, xenograft, and GTR. *Int. J. Periodontics Restor. Dent.* **2004**, *24*, 326–333.
63. Sculean, A.; Donos, N.; Schwarz, F.; Becker, J.; Brecx, M.; Arweiler, N.B. Five-year results following treatment of intrabony defects with enamel matrix proteins and guided tissue regeneration. *J. Clin. Periodontol.* **2004**, *31*, 545–549. [CrossRef] [PubMed]
64. Sculean, A.; Schwarz, F.; Miliauskaite, A.; Kiss, A.; Arweiler, N.; Becker, J.; Brecx, M. Treatment of intrabony defects with an enamel matrix protein derivative or bioabsorbable membrane: An 8-year follow-up split-mouth study. *J. Periodontol.* **2006**, *77*, 1879–1886. [CrossRef] [PubMed]
65. Sculean, A.; Schwarz, F.; Chiantella, G.C.; Arweiler, N.B.; Becker, J. Nine-year results following treatment of intrabony periodontal defects with an enamel matrix derivative: Report of 26 cases. *Int. J. Periodontics Restor. Dent.* **2007**, *27*, 221–229.
66. Sculean, A.; Kiss, A.; Miliauskaite, A.; Schwarz, F.; Arweiler, N.B.; Hannig, M. Ten-year results following treatment of intra-bony defects with enamel matrix proteins and guided tissue regeneration. *J. Clin. Periodontol.* **2008**, *35*, 817–824. [CrossRef] [PubMed]
67. Tonetti, M.S.; Lang, N.P.; Cortellini, P.; Suvan, J.E.; Adriaens, P.; Dubravec, D.; Fonzar, A.; Fourmousis, I.; Mayfield, L.; Rossi, R.; et al. A systematic review of graft materials and biological agents for periodontal intraosseous defects. *J. Clin. Periodontol.* **2002**, *3*, 117–135.

68. Windisch, P.; Sculean, A.; Klein, F.; Tóth, V.; Gera, I.; Reich, E.; Eickholz, P. Comparison of clinical, radiographic, and histometric measurements following treatment with guided tissue regeneration or enamel matrix proteins in human periodontal defects. *J. Periodontol.* **2002**, *73*, 409–417. [CrossRef]
69. Sanz, M.; Tonetti, M.S.; Zabalegui, I.; Sicilia, A.; Blanco, J.; Rebelo, H.; Rasperini, G.; Merli, M.; Cortellini, P.; Suvan, J.E. Treatment of intrabony defects with enamel matrix proteins or barrier membranes: Results from a multicenter practice-based clinical trial. *J. Periodontol.* **2004**, *75*, 726–733. [CrossRef]
70. Cortellini, P.; Tonetti, M.S. Clinical performance of a regenerative strategy for intrabony defects: Scientific evidence and clinical experience. *J. Periodontol.* **2005**, *76*, 341–350. [CrossRef]
71. Esposito, M.; Grusovin, M.G.; Papanikolaou, N.; Coulthard, P.; Worthington, H.V. Enamel matrix derivative (Emdogain) for periodontal tissue regeneration in intrabony defects. A Cochrane systematic review. *Eur. J. Oral Implantol.* **2009**, *2*, 247–266. [PubMed]
72. Koop, R.; Merheb, J.; Quirynen, M. Periodontal regeneration with enamel matrix derivative in reconstructive periodontal therapy: A systematic review. *J. Periodontol.* **2012**, *83*, 707–720. [CrossRef] [PubMed]
73. Döri, F.; Arweiler, N.B.; Szántó, E.; Agics, A.; Gera, I.; Sculean, A. Ten-year results following treatment of intrabony defects with an enamel matrix protein derivative combined with either a natural bone mineral or a β-tricalcium phosphate. *J. Periodontol.* **2013**, *84*, 749–757. [CrossRef] [PubMed]
74. Vandana, K.L.; Shah, K.; Prakash, S. Clinical and radiographic evaluation of Emdogain as a regenerative material in the treatment of interproximal vertical defects in chronic and aggressive periodontitis patients. *Int. J. Periodontics Restor. Dent.* **2004**, *24*, 185–191.
75. DiBattista, P.; Bissada, N.F.; Ricchetti, P.A. Comparative effectiveness of various regenerative modalities for the treatment of localized juvenile periodontitis. *J. Periodontol.* **1995**, *66*, 673–678. [CrossRef] [PubMed]
76. Palmer, R.M.; Cortellini, P. Group B of European Workshop on Periodontology Periodontal tissue engineering and regeneration: Consensus Report of the Sixth European Workshop on Periodontology. *J. Clin. Periodontol.* **2008**, *35*, 83–86. [CrossRef] [PubMed]
77. Rescala, B.; Rosalem, W., Jr.; Teles, R.P.; Fischer, R.G.; Haffajee, A.D.; Socransky, S.S.; Gustafsson, A.; Figueredo, C.M. Immunologic and microbiologic profiles of chronic and aggressive periodontitis subjects. *J. Periodontol.* **2010**, *81*, 1308–1316. [CrossRef]
78. Rosalem, W.; Rescala, B.; Teles, R.P.; Fischer, R.G.; Gustafsson, A.; Figueredo, C.M. Effect of non-surgical treatment on chronic and aggressive periodontitis: Clinical, immunologic, and microbiologic findings. *J. Periodontol.* **2011**, *82*, 979–989. [CrossRef]
79. Sant'Ana, A.C.; Passanezi, E.; Todescan, S.M.; de Rezende, M.L.; Greghi, S.L.; Ribeiro, M.G. A combined regenerative approach for the treatment of aggressive periodontitis: Long-term follow-up of a familial case. *Int. J. Periodontics Restor. Dent.* **2009**, *29*, 69–79.
80. Lu, R.F.; Xu, L.; Meng, H.X.; Feng, X.H.; Liu, K.N. Treatment of generalized aggressive periodontitis: A 4-year follow-up case report. *Chinese J. Dent. Res.* **2012**, *15*, 61–67.
81. Manor, A. Periodontal regeneration with enamel matrix derivative—Case reports. *J. Int. Acad. Periodontol.* **2000**, *2*, 44–48. [PubMed]
82. Stavropoulos, A.; Karring, T. Five-year results of guided tissue regeneration in combination with deproteinized bovine bone (Bio-Oss) in the treatment of intrabony periodontal defects: A case series report. *Clin. Oral Investig.* **2005**, *9*, 271–277. [CrossRef] [PubMed]
83. Lekovic, V.; Camargo, P.M.; Weinlaender, M.; Vasilic, N.; Djordjevic, M.; Kenney, E.B. The use of bovine porous bone mineral in combination with enamel matrix proteins or with an autologous fibrinogen/fibronectin system in the treatment of intrabony periodontal defects in humans. *J. Periodontol.* **2001**, *72*, 1157–1163. [CrossRef] [PubMed]
84. Lindhe, J.; Cecchinato, D.; Donati, M.; Tomasi, C.; Liljenberg, B. Ridge preservation with the use of deproteinized bovine bone mineral. *Clin. Oral Implants Res.* **2014**, *25*, 786–790. [CrossRef] [PubMed]

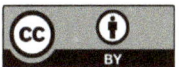 © 2019 by the authors. Licensee MDPI, Basel, Switzerland. This article is an open access article distributed under the terms and conditions of the Creative Commons Attribution (CC BY) license (http://creativecommons.org/licenses/by/4.0/).

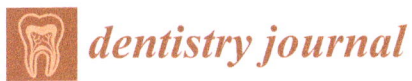

Article

Spectrophotometric Determination of the Aggregation Activity of Platelets in Platelet-Rich Plasma for Better Quality Control

Tetsuhiro Tsujino [1], Kazushige Isobe [1], Hideo Kawabata [1], Hachidai Aizawa [1], Sadahiro Yamaguchi [1], Yutaka Kitamura [1], Hideo Masuki [1], Taisuke Watanabe [1], Hajime Okudera [1], Koh Nakata [2] and Tomoyuki Kawase [3,*]

[1] Tokyo Plastic Dental Society, Kita-ku, Tokyo 114-0002, Japan; tetsudds@gmail.com (T.T.); kaz-iso@tc4.so-net.ne.jp (K.I.); hidei@eos.ocn.ne.jp (H.K.); sarusaru@mx6.mesh.ne.jp (H.A.); y-sada@mwd.biglobe.ne.jp (S.Y.); shinshu-osic@mbn.nifty.com (Y.K.); hideomasuki@gmail.com (H.M.); watatai@mui.biglobe.ne.jp (T.W.); okudera@carrot.ocn.ne.jp (H.O.)

[2] Bioscience Medical Research Center, Niigata University Medical and Dental Hospital, Niigata 951-8520, Japan; radical@med.niigata-u.ac.jp

[3] Division of Oral Bioengineering, Institute of Medicine and Dentistry, Niigata University, Niigata 951-8514, Japan

* Correspondence: kawase@dent.niigata-u.ac.jp; Tel.: +81-25-262-7559

Received: 28 April 2019; Accepted: 30 May 2019; Published: 3 June 2019

Abstract: Although platelet-rich plasma (PRP) is now widely used in regenerative medicine and dentistry, contradictory clinical outcomes have often been obtained. To minimize such differences and to obtain high quality evidence from clinical studies, the PRP preparation protocol needs to be standardized. In addition, emphasis must be placed on quality control. Following our previous spectrophotometric method of platelet counting, in this study, another simple and convenient spectrophotometric method to determine platelet aggregation activity has been developed. Citrated blood samples were collected from healthy donors and used. After centrifugation twice, platelets were suspended in phosphate buffered saline (PBS) and adenosine diphosphate (ADP)-induced aggregation was determined using a spectrophotometer at 615 nm. For validation, platelets pretreated with aspirin, an antiplatelet agent, or hydrogen peroxide (H_2O_2), an oxidative stress-inducing agent, were also analyzed. Optimal platelet concentration, assay buffer solution, and representative time point for determination of aggregation were found to be 50–$100 \times 10^4/\mu L$, PBS, and 3 min after stimulation, respectively. Suppressed or injured platelets showed a significantly lower aggregation response to ADP. Therefore, it suggests that this spectrophotometric method may be useful in quick chair-side evaluation of individual PRP quality.

Keywords: platelet-rich plasma; platelets; aggregation; spectrophotometer; quality assurance

1. Introduction

Since the first report by Marx et al. [1], regenerative therapy using platelet-rich plasma (PRP) has been increasingly used as a promising therapeutic method for more than two decades. However, in several tissues, such as bone, PRP therapy has not produced positive clinical outcomes. Differences in bone regeneration have been thought to mainly be because of individual differences in blood samples. Few efforts to overcome this hurdle have been made at the national and international levels. As a result, clear and strong evidence on the use of PRP, which can be adopted by individual national regulatory agencies and thereby support the clinical use of PRP, has not yet been obtained [2].

It could be argued that such differences could be eliminated by increasing the sample size. However, in the case of home-made PRP, prepared at the time of use, quality cannot be controlled or assured like factory-made products. Differences in individual PRP preparations are also due to the different preparation protocols, devices, and operator skills. Without careful consideration of the mentioned technical biases, reliable randomized clinical trials cannot be initiated for PRP therapy. Despite this situation, a recent proposal to standardize the PRP preparation protocol is expected to improve the quality of clinical evidence. Furthermore, sharing the concept of "quality control" among individual clinicians will complement the current standardization movement to assure similarity in the quality of individual PRP preparations in the near future.

In general, the quality of the cell-based medicinal products (CBMPs) is defined and evaluated mainly based on the following five parameters: sterility, purity, identity, potency, and stability [3]. However, home-made PRP is distinguished from the typical CBMP, such as hematopoietic stem cells, due to various factors. PRP quality can be defined by platelet count, growth factors present and their levels, coagulation activity, and platelet activity. Contamination with leukocytes might be an additional parameter influencing the quality [4,5]. It is not easy to determine platelet and leukocyte counts without using an automated hematology analyzer, which cannot be easily installed in dental clinics due to high initial investment and space required. Therefore, in a previous study [6], a simple and convenient assay method to quickly determine the platelet count using a pocketable spectrophotometer was developed. Coagulation activity is routinely determined by pocketable machines, e.g., CoaguChek® XS Plus (Roche, Basel, Switzerland). Thus, assays to rapidly determine the growth factor levels and platelet activity need to be developed.

This study focuses on platelet aggregation activity as a representative of platelet function. Moreover, it focuses on a microplate-reader-based technology to evaluate platelet aggregation as an alternative to the conventional type of aggregometer [7–10]. According to this principle, we have developed a spectrophotometric assay to evaluate adenosine diphosphate (ADP)-induced platelet aggregation in a quantitative manner. The primary purpose of this study was to test our modified spectrophotometric assay for platelet aggregation. The secondary purpose was to validate this assay method to evaluate the quality of platelets contained in individual PRP preparations by establishing the reference range and improving the quality of clinical evidence in cooperation with other assay methods. We successfully validated the assay's applicability by comparing normal platelets with suppressed and injured platelets. Although this study was limited by the size and variation of samples, we successfully optimized the assay conditions and suggest its applicability in quality control of individual PRP preparations.

2. Materials and Methods

2.1. Preparation of P-PRP and Platelet Suspension

Blood samples were collected from 14 healthy, nonsmoking adult volunteers in the age group of 22 to 70 (Male: N = 11, mean = 51.5 y, Female: N = 3, mean = 25.3 y) using butterfly needles (21G × $\frac{3}{4}$ in.; NIPRO, Osaka, Japan). Despite having lifestyle-related diseases and taking medication, these donors had no limitations on the activities of daily living. These donors also declared to be free of Human immunodeficiency virus (HIV), Hepatitis B virus (HBV), Hepatitis C virus (HCV), or syphilis infections. In addition, a prothrombin test was performed on all the blood samples by means of CoaguChek® XS, and all the samples were found to be normal in blood cell counts.

Peripheral blood samples (~7 mL) were collected into plastic vacuum plain blood collection tubes (Neotube; NIPRO, Osaka, Japan) containing 1 mL of acid–citrate–dextrose formula A (ACD-A; Terumo, Tokyo, Japan). Fresh whole-blood samples were immediately centrifuged at 530× g for 10 min or stored for up to 2 days before centrifugation at ambient temperature [11,12]. The upper plasma fraction, known as the platelet-rich plasma (PRP) fraction, was collected, transferred into fresh sample tubes, and treated for 10 min with 1 µg/mL prostaglandin E_1 (PGE_1; Cayman Chemical, Ann Arbor, MI, USA) [13,14]. The PRP fraction was again centrifuged at 2650× g for 3 min. Precipitated platelets were gently resuspended in acellular plasma, Tyrode buffer solution, phosphate buffered saline (PBS) or PBS containing ethylenediaminetetraacetic acid (EDTA) (final concentration: approximately 1.5 mg/mL). The platelet suspension in acellular plasma was designated as "pure PRP (P-PRP)." The number of platelets and other blood cells within the whole-blood samples and platelet suspensions was determined using an automated hematology analyzer (pocH 100iV, Sysmex, Kobe, Japan).

The study design and consent forms for all the procedures (project identification code: 2297) were approved by the Ethics Committee for Human Subjects of the Niigata University School of Medicine (Niigata, Japan) on 14 October 2015, in accordance with the Helsinki Declaration of 1964 as revised in 2013.

2.2. Spectrophotometric Determination of Platelet Aggregation

P-PRP and other platelet suspensions were serially diluted with equal volume of acellular plasma or the corresponding buffer solutions. Series of diluted platelet suspensions were measured using a pocketable spectrophotometer (PiCOSCOPE, Ushio Inc., Tokyo, Japan) [6]. The spectrophotometer can be operated by remote control through a specific application installed on smart devices, including the iPad Air (Apple, Cupertino, CA, USA). Platelet suspensions were transferred into 0.2 mL highly transparent PCR tubes (Nippon Genetics Co., Ltd., Tokyo, Japan) and treated with 5 µM ADP (Wako Pure Chemicals, Osaka, Japan).

To prepare dysfunctional platelet models, we pretreated P-PRP with 0.1 mg/mL aspirin (acetylsalicylic acid; Wako Pure Chemicals, Osaka, Japan) or 10 µM H_2O_2 (Wako) for 30 min at 22–24 °C. The absorbance was measured at an interval of one minute at 615 nm (range of wavelength: 570–660 nm). At the end of measurement, each blank was measured as the absorbance of 100% aggregation.

2.3. Statistical Analysis

Data were expressed as mean ± standard deviation (SD) or box plot (Figure 1). For multigroup comparisons, statistical analyses were performed to compare the mean values by Kruskal–Wallis one-way analysis of variance, followed by Steel–Dwass multiple comparison test (BellCurve for Excel; Social Survey Research Information Co., Ltd., Tokyo, Japan). Differences with $p < 0.05$ were considered statistically significant.

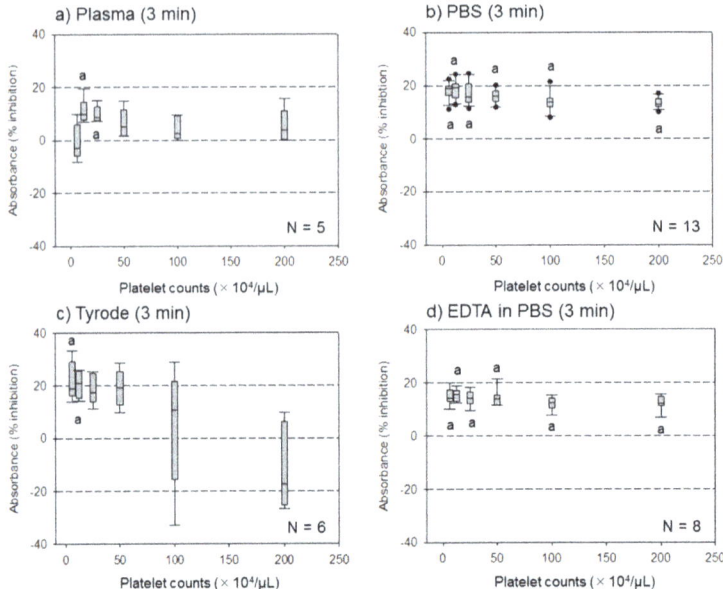

Figure 1. Effects of different assay buffer solutions on the adenosine diphosphate (ADP)-induced platelet aggregation. Platelets were suspended in (**a**) acellular plasma, (**b**) phosphate buffered saline (PBS), (**c**) Tyrode buffer solution, or (**d**) ethylenediaminetetraacetic acid (EDTA)-containing PBS at the indicated densities and stimulated with 5 μM ADP for 3 min at 22–24 °C. ^{a} $p < 0.05$ compared with individual corresponding controls at 0 min.

3. Results

3.1. Effect of Different Assay Buffer Solutions, Time Points, and Platelet Densities on the Assay System

The effect of different assay buffer solutions on the ADP-induced platelet aggregation assessed by the assay system at 3 min is shown in Figure 1. For platelets suspended in acellular plasma, the percentage inhibition levels were lower than those of others, based on the platelet density tested. However, the effects of ADP were sustained at lower platelet densities for platelets suspended in the Tyrode buffer solution. In contrast, for the platelets suspended in PBS and EDTA-containing PBS, the effects of ADP were constantly sustained between approximately 15%–20%, which was in the range of the platelet densities tested.

The effect of platelet density on ADP-induced platelet aggregation over a time course as assessed by the assay system is shown in Figure 2. Generally, platelets suspended in Tyrode buffer solution showed a better response to ADP because of the presence of Ca^{2+}; however, as the platelet density increased, the platelets tended to aggregate in this solution. In about a half of the samples, we found macroscopically identifiable platelet aggregates immediately after suspension in this solution. We did not use these suspensions for data collection, since the platelet number could not be counted. In contrast, platelets in PBS and EDTA-containing PBS responded similarly to ADP, although an increase in the platelet density slightly reduced platelet responsiveness (i.e., percentage inhibition).

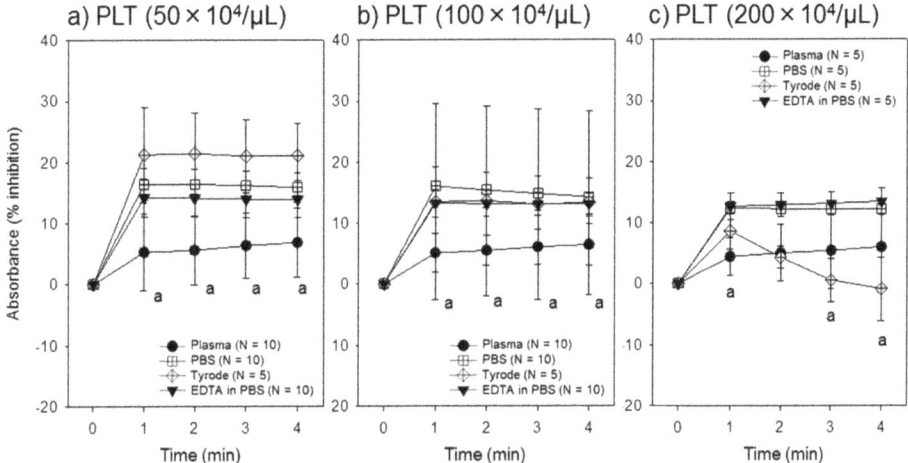

Figure 2. Effect of platelet density on ADP-induced platelet aggregation over a time course. Platelets were suspended in acellular plasma, PBS, Tyrode buffer solution, or EDTA-containing PBS at a density of (**a**) $50 \times 10^4/\mu L$, (**b**) $100 \times 10^4/\mu L$ or (**c**) $200 \times 10^4/\mu L$ and stimulated with 5 µM ADP for up to 4 min at 22–24 °C. [a] $p < 0.05$ compared with the data of PBS at the same time points.

3.2. Effect of Different Platelet Conditions on the Assay System

The effect of platelet condition on ADP-induced platelet aggregation assessed by the assay system at 3 min is shown in Figure 3. Except at lower platelet densities, the base line was stable and sustained at similar levels. Response to ADP was significantly reduced in platelets suppressed by aspirin and injured by H_2O_2.

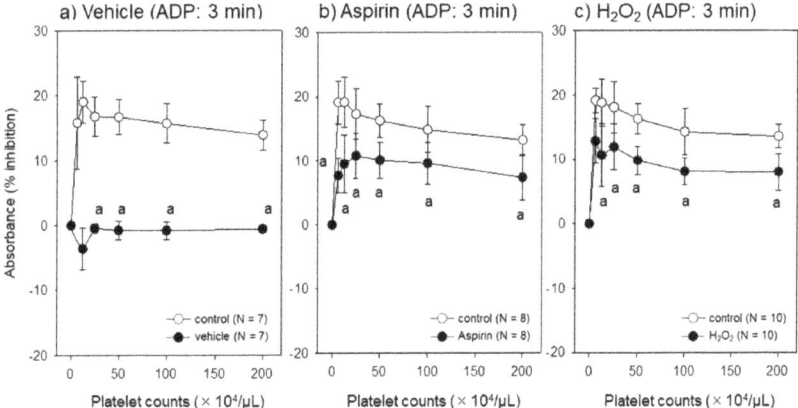

Figure 3. Effect of different platelet conditions on the ADP-induced platelet aggregations. Platelets suspended in acellular plasma were treated with (**a**) a vehicle of aspirin (0.1% dimethyl sulfoxide), (**b**) aspirin or (**c**) H_2O_2 for 30 min prior to resuspension in PBS and were stimulated with 5 µM ADP for 3 min. (**a**) The base line was monitored with no addition. [a] $p < 0.05$ compared with the control at the same platelet densities.

The effect of platelet density on ADP-induced aggregation of dysfunctional platelets over a time course assessed by the assay system is shown in Figure 4. Regardless of platelet density, both aspirin and H_2O_2 significantly reduced platelet responsiveness to ADP. However, it should be noted that at a higher platelet density, the degree of reduction apparently decreased.

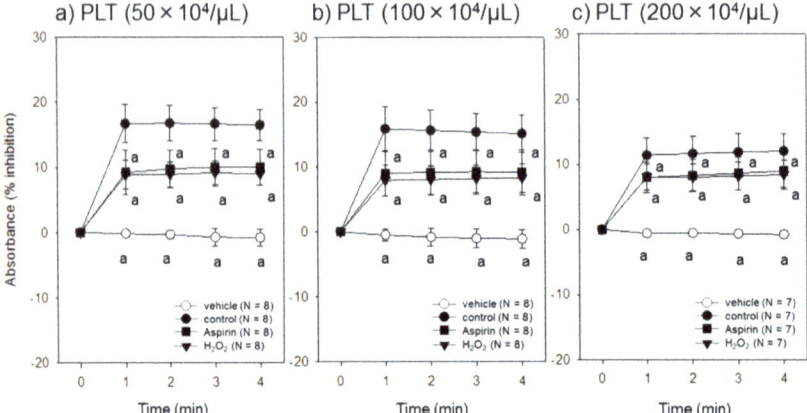

Figure 4. Effect of platelet densities on ADP-induced aggregation of dysfunctional platelets over a time course. Platelets were treated with a vehicle of aspirin (0.1% dimethyl sulfoxide), aspirin or H_2O_2, resuspended in PBS at a density of (**a**) $50 \times 10^4/\mu L$, (**b**) $100 \times 10^4/\mu L$ or (**c**) $200 \times 10^4/\mu L$ and stimulated with 5 µM ADP for up to 4 min at ambient temperature. ^{a} $p < 0.05$ compared with the corresponding controls at the same time points.

4. Discussion

In this study, we used blood samples collected from healthy donors who did not receive any medication and stored them for up to 2 days prior to preparation of pure PRP (P-PRP). After double centrifugation, platelets were resuspended in PBS and stimulated with ADP. Our spectrophotometric assay method demonstrated that these platelets responded to ADP similarly regardless of individual differences. After 3 min of stimulation, although the platelet count slightly increased, the absorbance (raw value) decreased by 10%–20% in response to ADP. Moreover, we also found that platelets treated with aspirin or H_2O_2 showed significantly reduced responsiveness to ADP.

These observations are further analyzed in detail below. To optimize the analysis conditions, we focused on (1) assay buffer solutions, (2) a range of platelet densities and (3) end points for data collection. In addition, to validate this method, we developed and examined (4) models of partially dysfunctional platelets using aspirin and H_2O_2.

4.1. Optimal Assay Buffer Solutions

In a previous study [6], based on handling efficiency, we chose acellular plasma to prepare platelet suspensions, i.e., P-PRP, and validated the applicability of the spectrophotometric method to determine platelet count. The plasma was a good "buffer solution" that could be used to easily and efficiently suspend precipitated platelets. However, in this study, we showed that although PRP is the recommended type of platelet suspension for aggregometric assays [15], plasma substantially reduced ADP-induced platelet aggregation. This is probably due to ectonucleotidases and/or similar enzymes present in the plasma, which quickly degrade ADP. Alternatively, certain plasma proteins, such as albumin, may block contact between ADP and its specific platelet receptors.

It is known that Ca^{2+} plays a crucial role in maintaining platelet functions, such as aggregation. Thus, we analyzed the effects of the Ca^{2+} and Mg^{2+}-containing Tyrode buffer solution as an alternative to plasma, because this buffer has been frequently used in the conventional assay involving a platelet aggregometer. However, the Tyrode buffer induced platelet aggregation at high rates in our experimental system, especially in the case of freshly prepared P-PRP, even though prostaglandin E_1

(PGE$_1$) was added to P-PRP prior to suspending platelets in the Tyrode buffer. Thus, we chose PBS to investigate the Ca^{2+}-induced platelet activation and morphological changes, as in our previous studies [16,17].

We then examined Ca^{2+}, and Mg^{2+}-free PBS and added EDTA to further eliminate the divalent cations. In general, PBS enabled suspension of precipitated platelets more efficiently than Tyrode buffer solution. In case of freshly prepared P-PRP, addition of EDTA caused efficient suspension of platelets in PBS without forming aggregates and sacrificing platelet responsiveness. This was confirmed by macroscopic examination and platelet counts. However, the superior effects of EDTA were not observed for blood samples stored over 2 h.

Also considering its low cost, high efficiency, and easy availability, we concluded that PBS can be used in a chair-side spectrophotometric assay for platelet aggregation.

4.2. Optimal Range of Platelet Density

Light transmission was examined through the bottom of the PCR sample tubes in this spectrophotometer. When platelet density was relatively low, the corresponding absorbance tended to increase gradually with gravity-dependent platelet sedimentation. This tendency could be counteracted by increased platelet density in a limited period of time. In contrast, when platelet densities were relatively high, platelet aggregation occurred, and no increase in absorbance was seen. This phenomenon may lead to underestimation of platelet activity. Therefore, we concluded that the optimal range of platelet density is roughly 50–100 × 10^4/µL.

4.3. Optimal End Point

Aggregation of human platelets in vitro can occur in two phases—primary and secondary aggregation [18]. With the pocketable spectrophotometer, we could not monitor changes in absorbance continuously; thus, we could not identify the pattern of aggregation through our assay system. The change in absorbance usually plateaued within 1–2 min and apparent additional changes did not occur within 5 min after stimulation. Therefore, any time point after 1 min of stimulation may be acceptable as an end point. Considering handling efficiency and probability of misoperation, we chose 3 min as an end point.

4.4. Comparisons with Suppressed or Injured Platelets

Under the mentioned optimal conditions, normal platelets were compared with artificially modified platelets. Aspirin is a conventional antiplatelet agent that inhibits cyclooxygenase-1, which forms thromboxane A$_2$ in response to secreted dense granule constituents, such as serotonin and ADP, in the secondary wave [18]. Thus, platelets treated with aspirin were expected to show reduced aggregation activity in response to ADP. We observed only approximately 50% inhibition when P-PRP was treated with 0.1 mg/mL aspirin for 20 min. Modification of the timing (from P-PRP to platelet suspension in PBS), duration (from 20 min to overnight), and concentration (from 0.1 mg/mL to 0.3 mg/mL) of aspirin did not significantly augment the inhibition. However, these findings indicate that the assay method is capable of distinguishing suppressed platelets from normal platelets.

Endogenously generated H$_2$O$_2$ is thought to function as a trigger for platelet activation and aggregation [19,20]. On the contrary, exogenously added H$_2$O$_2$, which is known as an inducer of oxidative stress, damages the plasma membrane through lipid peroxidation and alters fluidity and leakiness of the membrane. As a result, H$_2$O$_2$ inhibits ADP-dependent platelet activation [21]. In this study, as observed with aspirin, H$_2$O$_2$ inhibited ADP-induced platelet aggregation by approximately 50%. Thus, this suggests that when platelets are damaged by manual error during preparation or donor-dependent oxidative stress, this assay method is capable of indicating reduced PRP quality.

4.5. Limitations of This Study

Platelet aggregation activity assessed by conventional aggregometry is expressed by qualitative or semi-qualitative data. Unlike the platelet count, such data cannot be easily used for comparison with data from other samples. Moreover, Chandrashekar [22] mentioned that light transmission aggregometry lacks standardization and normal reference values are not widely available. However, our findings indicate the possibility that this simple and quick assay method could be used to assure individual PRP quality. At the same time, we should consider the limitations of this study, which could cause biases that lead to misinterpretation of the data.

ADP is one of the most important mediators of hemostasis and thrombosis, and thus has been used in conventional clinical laboratory testing of platelet function [23]. In addition, because of its simple chemical constitution, we chose ADP for the development of the assay method. The concern regarding the suitability of the aggregation assay in the assessment of PRP quality can be explained as follows. Since clot formation of PRP is induced by coagulation factors, such as thrombin or $CaCl_2$, or contact with glass surface in the presence of Ca^{2+}, it is obvious that platelets are activated primarily by thrombin and fibrin, but not by ADP. However, growth factor secretion, which is related to the most important criterion of PRP quality, and aggregation are simultaneous coupling events of activated platelets. Therefore, we thought that even with variations in the manners and/or degrees of platelet activation with individual meditators, ADP is acceptable for preparation of the basic model of activated platelets.

On the other hand, this study was done using a small sample size consisting of volunteers of Japanese ethnicity. Therefore, individual differences are relatively lower and we may have obtained statistical significances in ADP-induced aggregation between control platelets and the dysfunctional ones. However, recent advances in platelet studies have revealed that platelet functions, which include responses to ADP and sensitivity to aspirin, vary qualitatively and quantitatively with genetic differences among races and individuals [23–26]. To efficiently detect inherited platelet disorders or dysfunctional platelets by reducing possible quantitative variations, we performed the assay with ADP at a concentration higher than the endogenous levels and aspirin at a concentration higher than the therapeutic levels. We concluded that these choices were optimal for our samples.

However, to realize this assay method as a globally standardized protocol for assessment of PRP quality in regenerative dentistry, further verification and subsequent improvement should be done with larger sample sizes by organizing international round robin testing. In addition, to evaluate PRP quality comprehensively in a timely manner, this kind of platelet function testing should be done with other tests regarding growth factor levels, platelet counts, and coagulation activity.

5. Conclusions

Our assay method, developed to evaluate platelet aggregation activity, is simple, quick, and sensitive enough to detect dysfunctional platelets. In addition, this method does not require high initial investment, technical training, or space in clinics. At present, we have no evidence that platelet aggregation activity influences PRP clinical efficiency; however, this assay method, in combination with other assay methods and standardization of preparation protocols, will enable assurance of individual PRP quality and facilitate high quality randomized controlled trials to obtain strong evidence in support of PRP therapy. This will further aid in terminating the current endless debate on PRP efficiency.

Author Contributions: Conceptualization, T.T. and T.K.; methodology, T.K.; validation, T.T. and K.I.; formal analysis, T.T. and T.K.; investigation, T.T., K.I., H.K., H.A., S.Y., Y.K. and H.M. and T.W.; resources, T.T. and K.I.; data curation, Y.K., H.O. and K.N.; Writing—Original Draft preparation, T.T. and T.K.; Writing—Review and Editing, T.T., K.I. and T.K.; visualization, T.K.; supervision, H.O. and K.N.; project administration, T.W. and T.K.; funding acquisition, T.K.

Funding: This research was funded in part by JSPS KAKENHI (Grant Number 18K09595).

Conflicts of Interest: The authors declare no conflict of interest.

Abbreviations

PRP	Platelet-rich plasma
P-PRP	Pure platelet-rich plasma
ACD-A	Acid-citrate-dextrose formula A
ADP	Adenosine diphosphate
PGE_1	Prostaglandin E_1
PBS	Phosphate buffered saline
PCR	Polymerase chain reaction
H_2O_2	Hydrogen peroxide
EDTA	Ethylenediaminetetraacetic acid
CBMP	Cell-based medicinal product
HIV	Human immunodeficiency virus
HBV	Hepatitis B virus
HCV	Hepatitis C virus

References

1. Marx, R.E.; Carlson, E.R.; Eichstaedt, R.M.; Schimmele, S.R.; Strauss, J.E.; Georgeff, K.R. Platelet-rich plasma: Growth factor enhancement for bone grafts. *Oral Surg. Oral Med. Oral Pathol. Oral Radiol. Endodontol.* **1998**, *85*, 638–646. [CrossRef]
2. Kawase, T.; Takahashi, A.; Watanabe, T.; Tsujino, T. Proposal for point-of-care testing of platelet-rich plasma quality. *Int. J. Growth Factors Stem Cells Dent.* **2019**, *2*, 13–17. [CrossRef]
3. Kawase, T.; Okuda, K. Comprehensive Quality Control of the Regenerative Therapy Using Platelet Concentrates: The Current Situation and Prospects in Japan. *BioMed Res. Int.* **2018**, *2018*, 6389157. [CrossRef]
4. Anitua, E.; Zalduendo, M.; Troya, M.; Padilla, S.; Orive, G. Leukocyte inclusion within a platelet rich plasma-derived fibrin scaffold stimulates a more pro-inflammatory environment and alters fibrin properties. *PLoS ONE* **2015**, *10*, e0121713. [CrossRef] [PubMed]
5. Xu, Z.; Yin, W.; Zhang, Y.; Qi, X.; Chen, Y.; Xie, X.; Zhang, C. Comparative evaluation of leukocyte- and platelet-rich plasma and pure platelet-rich plasma for cartilage regeneration. *Sci. Rep.* **2017**, *7*, 43301. [CrossRef] [PubMed]
6. Kitamura, Y.; Suzuki, M.; Tsukioka, T.; Isobe, K.; Tsujino, T.; Watanabe, T.; Watanabe, T.; Okudera, H.; Nakata, K.; Tanaka, T.; et al. Spectrophotometric determination of platelet counts in platelet-rich plasma. *Int. J. Implant Dent.* **2018**, *4*, 29. [CrossRef]
7. Bednar, B.; Condra, C.; Gould, R.J.; Connolly, T.M. Platelet aggregation monitored in a 96 well microplate reader is useful for evaluation of platelet agonists and antagonists. *Thromb. Res.* **1995**, *77*, 453–463. [CrossRef]
8. Chan, M.V.; Armstrong, P.C.; Warner, T.D. 96-well plate-based aggregometry. *Platelets* **2018**, *29*, 650–655. [CrossRef]
9. Krause, S.; Scholz, T.; Temmler, U.; Losche, W. Monitoring the effects of platelet glycoprotein IIb/IIIa antagonists with a microtiter plate method for detection of platelet aggregation. *Platelets* **2001**, *12*, 423–430. [CrossRef]
10. Fratantoni, J.C.; Poindexter, B.J. Measuring platelet aggregation with microplate reader. A new technical approach to platelet aggregation studies. *Am. J. Clin. Pathol.* **1990**, *94*, 613–617. [CrossRef]
11. Isobe, K.; Suzuki, M.; Watanabe, T.; Kitamura, Y.; Suzuki, T.; Kawabata, H.; Nakamura, M.; Okudera, T.; Okudera, H.; Uematsu, K.; et al. Platelet-rich fibrin prepared from stored whole-blood samples. *Int. J. Implant Dent.* **2017**, *3*, 6. [CrossRef] [PubMed]
12. Kawabata, H.; Isobe, K.; Watanabe, T.; Okudera, T.; Nakamura, M.; Suzuki, M.; Ryu, J.; Kitamura, Y.; Okudera, H.; Okuda, K.; et al. Quality Assessment of Platelet-Rich Fibrin-Like Matrix Prepared from Whole Blood Samples after Extended Storage. *Biomedicines* **2017**, *5*, 57. [CrossRef]
13. Takahashi, A.; Takahashi, S.; Tsujino, T.; Isobe, K.; Watanabe, T.; Kitamura, Y.; Watanabe, T.; Nakata, K.; Kawase, T. Platelet adhesion on commercially pure titanium plates in vitro I: Effects of plasma components and involvement of the von Willebrand factor and fibronectin. *Int. J. Implant Dent.* **2019**, *5*, 5. [CrossRef] [PubMed]

14. Watanabe, T.; Isobe, K.; Suzuki, T.; Kawabata, H.; Nakamura, M.; Tsukioka, T.; Okudera, T.; Okudera, H.; Uematsu, K.; Okuda, K.; et al. An Evaluation of the Accuracy of the Subtraction Method Used for Determining Platelet Counts in Advanced Platelet-Rich Fibrin and Concentrated Growth Factor Preparations. *Dent. J.* **2017**, *5*, 7. [CrossRef] [PubMed]
15. Practical-Haemostasis.com. A Practical Guide to Laboratory Haemostasis. Volume 2019. 2013. Available online: http://www.practical-haemostasis.com/Platelets/platelet_function_testing_lta.html (accessed on 16 April 2019).
16. Kitamura, Y.; Isobe, K.; Kawabata, H.; Tsujino, T.; Watanabe, T.; Nakamura, M.; Toyoda, T.; Okudera, H.; Okuda, K.; Nakata, K.; et al. Quantitative evaluation of morphological changes in activated platelets in vitro using digital holographic microscopy. *Micron* **2018**, *113*, 1–9. [CrossRef] [PubMed]
17. Toyoda, T.; Isobe, K.; Tsujino, T.; Koyata, Y.; Ohyagi, F.; Watanabe, T.; Nakamura, M.; Kitamura, Y.; Okudera, H.; Nakata, K.; et al. Direct activation of platelets by addition of $CaCl_2$ leads coagulation of platelet-rich plasma. *Int. J. Implant Dent.* **2018**, *4*, 23. [CrossRef]
18. Meyers, K.M.; Lindner, C.; Katz, J.; Grant, B. Phenylbutazone inhibition of equine platelet function. *Am. J. Vet. Res.* **1979**, *40*, 265–270. [PubMed]
19. Belisario, M.A.; Tafuri, S.; Di Domenico, C.; Squillacioti, C.; Della Morte, R.; Lucisano, A.; Staiano, N. H_2O_2 activity on platelet adhesion to fibrinogen and protein tyrosine phosphorylation. *Biochim. Biophys. Acta* **2000**, *1495*, 183–193. [CrossRef]
20. Del Principe, D.; Menichelli, A.; De Matteis, W.; Di Corpo, M.L.; Di Giulio, S.; Finazzi-Agro, A. Hydrogen peroxide has a role in the aggregation of human platelets. *FEBS Lett.* **1985**, *185*, 142–146. [CrossRef]
21. Krotz, F.; Sohn, H.Y.; Pohl, U. Reactive oxygen species: Players in the platelet game. *Arterioscler. Thromb. Vasc. Biol.* **2004**, *24*, 1988–1996. [CrossRef]
22. Chandrashekar, V. Does platelet count in platelet-rich plasma influence slope, maximal amplitude and lag phase in healthy individuals? Results of light transmission aggregometry. *Platelets* **2015**, *26*, 699–701. [CrossRef] [PubMed]
23. Lindkvist, M.; Fernberg, U.; Ljungberg, L.U.; Falker, K.; Fernstrom, M.; Hurtig-Wennlof, A.; Grenegard, M. Individual variations in platelet reactivity towards ADP, epinephrine, collagen and nitric oxide, and the association to arterial function in young, healthy adults. *Thromb. Res.* **2019**, *174*, 5–12. [CrossRef] [PubMed]
24. Backman, J.D.; Yerges-Armstrong, L.M.; Horenstein, R.B.; Newcomer, S.; Shaub, S.; Morrisey, M.; Donnelly, P.; Drolet, M.; Tanner, K.; Pavlovich, M.A.; et al. Prospective Evaluation of Genetic Variation in Platelet Endothelial Aggregation Receptor 1 Reveals Aspirin-Dependent Effects on Platelet Aggregation Pathways. *Clin. Transl. Sci.* **2017**, *10*, 102–109. [CrossRef] [PubMed]
25. Edelstein, L.C.; Simon, L.M.; Lindsay, C.R.; Kong, X.; Teruel-Montoya, R.; Tourdot, B.E.; Chen, E.S.; Ma, L.; Coughlin, S.; Nieman, M.; et al. Common variants in the human platelet PAR4 thrombin receptor alter platelet function and differ by race. *Blood* **2014**, *124*, 3450–3458. [CrossRef] [PubMed]
26. Fontana, P.; Dupont, A.; Gandrille, S.; Bachelot-Loza, C.; Reny, J.L.; Aiach, M.; Gaussem, P. Adenosine diphosphate-induced platelet aggregation is associated with P2Y12 gene sequence variations in healthy subjects. *Circulation* **2003**, *108*, 989–995. [CrossRef]

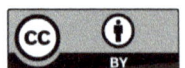

© 2019 by the authors. Licensee MDPI, Basel, Switzerland. This article is an open access article distributed under the terms and conditions of the Creative Commons Attribution (CC BY) license (http://creativecommons.org/licenses/by/4.0/).

MDPI
St. Alban-Anlage 66
4052 Basel
Switzerland
Tel. +41 61 683 77 34
Fax +41 61 302 89 18
www.mdpi.com

Dentistry Journal Editorial Office
E-mail: dentistry@mdpi.com
www.mdpi.com/journal/dentistry

www.ingramcontent.com/pod-product-compliance
Lightning Source LLC
LaVergne TN
LVHW072001080526
838202LV00064B/6810